Obstetric Anesthesia Pearls

William E. Ackerman • Mushtaque M. Juneja

William E. Ackerman III, MD
Associate Professor of Clinical Anesthesia
University of Cincinnati School of Medicine
Cincinnati, Ohio

Mushtaque M. Juneja, MD
Assistant Professor of Clinical Anesthesia
University of Cincinnati School of Medicine
Cincinnati, Ohio

APPLETON & LANGE
Norwalk, Connecticut/San Mateo, California

0-8385-7173-5

The authors and the publisher of this volume have taken care to make
certain that the doses of drugs and schedules of treatment are correct
and compatible with the standards generally accepted at the time of
publication. The reader is advised to consult carefully the instruction and
information material included in the package insert of each drug or
therapeutic agent before administration. This advice is especially important
when using new or infrequently used drugs.

Copyright © 1992 by Appleton & Lange
A Publishing Division of Prentice Hall

92 93 94 95 96 / 10 9 8 7 6 5 4 3 2 1

Prentice Hall International (UK) Limited, *London*
Prentice Hall of Australia Pty. Limited, *Sydney*
Prentice Hall of Canada Inc., *Toronto*
Prentice Hall Hispanoamericana, S.A., *Mexico*
Prentice Hall of India Private Limited, *New Delhi*
Prentice Hall of Japan, Inc., *Tokyo*
Prentice Hall of Southeast Asia Pte. Ltd., *Singapore*
Editora Prentice Hall do Brasil, Ltda., *Rio de Janeiro*
Prentice Hall, *Englewood Cliffs, New Jersey*

Library of Congress Cataloging-in-Publication Data

Ackerman, William E.
    Obstetric anesthesia pearls / William E. Ackerman III,
Mustaque M. Juneja.
        p.   cm.
    Includes index.
    ISBN (invalid) 0-8385-7173-5
    1. Anesthesia in obstetrics—Outlines, syllabi,
etc. I. Juneja, Mustaque M. II. Title.
    [DNLM: 1. Anesthesia, Obstetrical. 2. Delivery.
3. Labor. 4. Pregnancy Complications.   WO 450 A182o]
RG732.A3 1991
617.9′682—dc20
DNLM/DLC
for Library of Congress   91-4863
                                                 CIP

Acquisitions Editor: R. Craig Percy
Production Editor: Sandra K. Huggard
Designer: S.M. Byrum
PRINTED IN THE UNITED STATES OF AMERICA

Contents

Introduction

Obstetric Anesthesia Pearls was undertaken to provide anesthesia and obstetric practitioners with a concise synopsis of obstetric anesthesia. This book in its present format was requested by the anesthesia faculty, fellows, residents, medical students, CRNAs, and CRNA students at the University of Cincinnati Medical Center as well as private practitioners throughout the United States. It was written and developed while the authors were on the faculty at the University of Cincinnati. *Obstetric Anesthesia Pearls* was written with the assumption that the reader has some knowledge of the basic principles of regional and general anesthesia. With this in mind, *Obstetric Anesthesia Pearls* is intended to provide practitioners of obstetric anesthesia with a quick reference in an outline format that contains the information necessary for the management of common and not so common obstetric anesthesia problems. This manual is not intended to take the place of more comprehensive obstetric anesthesia textbooks, but is meant to provide the practitioner with a pocket reference of information while in attendance of the parturient.

We wish to thank Dr. Philip O. Bridenbaugh, Chairman of Anesthesiology at the University of Cincinnati, for his encouragement in the writing of this book. We further express our appreciation to Carolyn J.

Nicholson, CRNA, and Samina Juneja, MD for suggestions in the preparation of this manual, to Mary Ann Cost for her patience in typing this manual, and to Gretchen Ackerman, RN for her illustrations.

SECTION I

Fundamentals of Obstetric Anesthesia

1

Maternal Physiology

A thorough understanding of the physiological changes that occur during pregnancy is necessary when planning the administration of an anesthetic in the parturient.

I. Hematologic Changes

A. Blood volume: An increased blood volume is necessary to meet the metabolic needs of the fetus and to prepare the parturient for the blood loss encountered at delivery. The blood volume begins to increase after the eighth week and increases to approximately 40% above the prepregnancy values at term.

1. The red cell volume increases from 25 mL/kg to 30 mL/kg.
2. The plasma volume increases from 40 mL/kg to 70 mL/kg.
3. Clinically, the patient may appear anemic because the increase in plasma volume is greater than the increase in red cell mass. Anemia may be corrected by the administration of iron and folic acid.

B. Blood constituents
1. White blood cells
    a. In nonpregnant patients, the normal WBC is 5000 to 9000/mm^3.

    b. In pregnancy, the WBC increases to 15,000/mm^3.

    c. During labor, the WBC may increase to 25,000/mm^3.

2. The **platelets** remain normal during pregnancy.

3. The **plasma proteins** decrease due to a decrease in albumin (dilutional effect?).

4. Coagulation factors:
    a. In pregnancy, fibrinogen, prothrombin, factors VII, VIII, X, XII, and plasminogen are all elevated.

    b. Clinically, the increase in coagulant activity and the decrease in fibrinolysis make the pregnant patient more susceptible to thromboembolic phenomena. Essentially, the pregnant patient is hypercoagulable.

II. Cardiovascular Changes
A. Cardiac output
1. **During pregnancy,** the cardiac output increases during the first trimester and increases to approximately 30 to 40% over prepregnancy values at 28 to 32 weeks. The increase in cardiac output reflects an elevation of both the heart rate and blood volume.

2. During labor
    a. In the **latent** phase, there is a 15% increase in cardiac output.

    b. In the **active** phase, there is a 30% increase in cardiac output.

    c. In the **second stage** of labor, there is a 45% increase in cardiac output.

3. Postpartum, there is an 80% increase in cardiac output due to return of approximately 500 to 800 cc of blood into the central circulation after placental separation and myometrial contraction. These factors must be taken into consideration in patients with cardiac problems.

B. Vena caval compression

1. Vena caval compression is caused by the occlusion of the aorta and vena cava due to the gravid uterus (especially after 28 weeks) pressing against the vertebral column. It may cause a decreased venous return, stroke volume, and cardiac output in the pregnant woman. The total systemic vascular resistance (SVR) is decreased despite increases in plasma volume and increase in cardiac output. Only 10% of patients become symptomatic (hypotensive) because of insufficient collateral blood flow through the internal vertebral plexus. Occlusion of the lower aorta, which decreases uterine blood flow and placental perfusion, occurs much earlier (as early as 19 weeks) than occlusion of the upper aorta.

2. Clinical implications:

    a. A patient should not be supine beginning the second trimester of pregnancy. The patient should be placed in a left lateral tilt.

b. The uterus can be displaced from the great vessels by the use of a wedge or folded towel.

c. Venous engorgement of the internal vertebral plexus reduces the volumes of the epidural and subarachnoid spaces. Therefore, the dose of local anesthetic should be decreased by one third.

III. Respiratory Changes

A. Capillary engorgement of the respiratory tract produces a generalized redness and swelling.

1. If a nasal endotracheal tube must be used, it should be well lubricated and gently inserted to avoid the possibility of a nose bleed.

2. A smaller-sized endotracheal tube may be required for intubation because of swelling of the arytenoid region of the vocal cords in the pregnant patient.

B. Mechanical changes

1. The diaphragm is elevated 4 cm and is counterbalanced by an increase in the chest anteroposterior (AP) diameter.

2. With elevation of diaphragm, a 20% decrease in functional residual capacity (FRC) occurs, although total lung capacity remains unchanged. This decrease in FRC may lead to small-airway closure, especially in the obese parturient in the supine or lithotomy position.

C. Ventilation

1. Alveolar ventilation increases to approximately 70% above prepregnancy values at term due to an increase in tidal volume (TV) and an increase in respiratory rate. The increase in respiratory rate and tidal volume is caused by progesterone secretion.

2. Oxygen consumption increases 20%.

3. The arterial blood gases show compensated respiratory alkalosis:

   a. The PaO_2 is increased to 106 torr, or may be decreased.

   b. The $PaCO_2$ is decreased to 32 torr.

   c. The HCO_3 is decreased to 18 to 22 torr.

   d. The pH remains essentially unchanged.

4. **Minimal alveolar concentration** (MAC) is decreased in pregnancy.

5. **Clinical implications:**

   a. With a decrease in FRC, an increase in alveolar ventilation and an increase in oxygen consumption, the parturient is susceptible to hypoxemia. The pregnant patient should be preoxygenated to insure adequate denitrogenation before the induction of general anesthesia.

   b. Induction of general anesthesia and emergence will occur more rapidly in pregnant patients.

   c. A decreased MAC, decreased FRC, and increased alveolar ventilation predispose the parturient to anesthetic overdose.

IV. Gastrointestinal Changes

A. Mechanical changes

1. The position of the stomach shifts from a vertical to a horizontal plane.
2. The pylorus is pushed upward and backward.
3. A partial mechanical obstruction can occur, which can create an increase in intragastric pressure.
4. The gastric-emptying time is reduced.

B. Hormonal changes

1. Generalized smooth muscle relaxation occurs.
2. Increased gastric acidity is seen.
3. Delayed gastric emptying is seen.
4. A decreased lower esophageal sphincter tone (LES) is also noted.

C. Clinical implications

1. The parturient is susceptible to aspiration during the induction and emergence of general anesthesia.
2. All pregnant patients should be treated as having a full stomach regardless of when their last meal was ingested.
3. It has been suggested that a rapid sequence induction and intubation be performed during general anesthesia beginning in the second trimester or earlier if signs and symptoms of esophagitis are present.
4. Narcotics, diazepam, and atropine may all decrease lower esophageal sphincter tone and delay gastric emptying. The

routine administration of these drugs is not advocated. Furthermore, narcotics and diazepam can result in fetal depression.

5. Metoclopramide increases the lower esophageal tone and increases gastric emptying in some patients.

V. Renal Changes

A. Renal perfusion: The increase in blood volume causes a corresponding rise in renal plasma flow.

B. Glomerular filtration rate. The increase in renal plasma flow in turn increases glomerular filtration rate (GFR), thereby enhancing creatinine clearance.

C. Clinical implications

1. The creatinine, uric acid, and BUN lab values are normally lower in pregnant patients:

TEST	NONPREGNANT VALUE (mg%)	PREGNANT VALUE (mg%)
Creatinine	0.67 ± 0.14 (0.6–1.2)	0.46 ± 0.13
BUN	13 ± 3 (10–20)	8.5 ± 1.3
Uric acid	2.5–7.5	3.0–3.5

2. More water than sodium is retained during the third trimester of pregnancy, which causes the dependent edema of late pregnancy.

VI. Hepatic Changes

A. Plasma pseudocholinesterase levels are lower in pregnancy and immediately postpartum.

B. Clinical implications. Standard doses of succinylcholine do not produce problems.

However, one should use a nerve stimulator when using a succinylcholine infusion in order to minimize the incidence of a phase II blockade.

VII. Metabolic Changes

A. Alpha-fetoprotein levels are increased in chronic fetal distress, fetal death, and in normal multiple pregnancy. If the fetus has a neural tube defect or gastrointestinal tract obstruction, alpha fetoprotein may be increased in maternal plasma and in the amniotic fluid. Alpha fetoprotein is synthesized in the fetal liver and intestine.

B. Serum albumin levels decrease slightly and **serum globulin levels** increase slightly during pregnancy.

C. Carbohydrates metabolism. The pregnant patient is considered to be diabetogenic. Cellular sensitivity to insulin is reduced during pregnancy. Human chorionic somatotropin, however, increases peripheral use of glucose.

VIII. Hormonal Changes

A. Progesterone and estrogen levels are produced by the ovaries and exert physiological effects on the pregnant patient and are elevated during pregnancy.

1. Elevated progesterone levels produce the following:

   a. A decreased MAC due to progesterone's ability to produce somnolence.

   b. Hyperventilation manifested primarily as an increase in tidal volume.

   c. Increased body temperature and a

consequent increase in cutaneous perfusion to dissipate heat.

   d. A generalized decrease in smooth muscle tone may be seen resulting in relaxation of the gastroesophageal sphincter, decreased gastric empty-ing, constipation, and a dilated uterus.

2. Elevated estrogen levels produce the following:

   a. Nausea and vomiting in first trimes-ter.

   b. A hypercoagulable state due to in-creased clotting factors.

   c. An increased cardiac output and blood volume.

   d. An increased hepatic synthesis of an-giotensin and increased renin activity occur during pregnancy.

   e. An increased total serum protein oc-curs.

   f. Increased total lipid and fat deposi-tion also occurs.

   g. A positive nitrogen balance results from protein-sparing and anabolic ef-fects.

   h. The maintenance of the calcium bal-ance is maintained in the face of the large quantities of calcium demanded by fetal growth.

B. Anterior pituitary hormone levels

   1. Prolactin levels increase.

   2. The follicle-stimulating hormone and growth hormone levels decrease.

C. Posterior pituitary hormone levels remain unchanged.

D. Thyroid hormone levels
   1. The thyroid increases in size due to hyperplasia of glandular tissue and increased vascularity.
   2. The free T3 and T4 levels remain unchanged.
   3. The normal pregnant patient remains euthyroid throughout pregnancy.

E. Parathyroid hormone levels are increased.

F. Adrenal hormone levels. Estriol, estradiol, and estrane are increased, as are cortisol and corticosterone levels.

IX. Cutaneous Changes. Angiomas can develop on the upper part of the body. The midline of the abdomen may become pigmented.

X. Central Nervous System Changes. The parturient requires less local anesthetic because acid-base changes in the cerebrospinal fluid and hormonal changes increase nerve sensitivity to local anesthetics.

XI. Musculoskeletal Changes. Lordosis is characteristic of pregnancy. Low back pain and lower extremity weakness may be noted during the last trimester of pregnancy. Flexion of the neck can cause traction on the median and ulnar nerves of the upper extremities.

SUGGESTED READING

Crisp WE, DeFrancesco S. The hand syndrome of pregnancy. *Obstet Gynecol.* 1964; 23:433.

Datta S, Lambert DH, Gregus J et al. Differential sensitivities of mammalian nerve fibers during pregnancy. *Anesth Analg.* 1983; 62:1070.

Eckstein KL, Marx GF. Aortocaval compression and uterine displacement. *Anesthesiology.* 1974; 40:92.

Kerr M. Cardiovascular dynamics in pregnancy and labor. *Br Med Bull.* 1968; 24:19.

Lees MM, Taylor SH, Scott DB, et al. A study of cardiac output at rest throughout pregnancy. *J Obstet Gynecol Br Commonw.* 1967; 74:319.

Metcalf T, Ueland K. Maternal cardiovascular adjustments to pregnancy. *Prog Cardiovasc Dis.* 1974; 16:363.

Palahniuk RT, Shnider SM, Eger EI. II. Pregnancy decreases the requirements for inhaled anesthetic agents. *Anesthesiology.* 1974; 41:82.

Prowse CM, Gaensler EA. Respiratory and acid-base changes during pregnancy. *Anesthesiology.* 1965; 26:381.

2

Normal Labor and Labor Pain

Labor is a physiological process by which the fetus is expelled by the uterus. Labor occurs between 37 and 42 weeks from the last menstrual period.

  I. Stages of Labor

    A. The **first stage** of labor encompasses the interval of time from the onset of labor until the cervix becomes fully dilated (10 cm).

      1. The **latent phase** of the first stage is characterized by slow cervical dilation.

      2. The **active phase** of the first stage is characterized by a rapid cervical dilation.

    B. The **second stage** of labor begins with complete dilatation of the cervix and ends with delivery of the infant.

    C. The **third stage** of labor begins with delivery of the infant and ends with delivery of the placenta.

  II. Normal Duration of Labor

    A. First stage. The average rate of cervical dilatation in the active phase is 1.5 cm/hour in the multipara and 1.2 cm/hour in the nullipara patient. The latent phase may vary.

B. Second stage. The mean duration of the second stage is 20 minutes in multiparas and 50 minutes in the nullipara.

C. Third stage. The third stage of labor occurs within 1 to 5 minutes within delivery of the infant.

III. **Cardinal Movements of Labor in Normal Presentation**

A. Engagement. Descent of the biparietal plane of the fetal head below the pelvic inlet.

B. Descent. The first requisite for birth is descent, which is the entrance of the neonatal head into the pelvis.

C. Flexion. The chin is brought into contact with the fetal thorax.

D. Internal rotation. The occiput moves anteriorly to the symphysis pubis.

E. Extension. The base of the fetal occiput contacts the symphysis pubis.

F. External rotation. The head returns to the oblique position.

G. Expulsion. Extrusion of the infant from the vaginal vault.

IV. **Effects of Amniotomy on Progress of Labor**

An amniotomy is the artificial tearing of a hole in the membranes that the obstetrician performs for visualization of the amniotic fluid or for access for placement of an internal fetal monitor. It may hasten labor in some patients.

V. **Anesthetic Considerations Relating to Progress and Stage of Labor**

A. Epidural anesthesia has minimal to no effects on the progress of normal labor when the patient is in active labor provided that

severe prolonged hypotension is not permitted to occur.
B. Subarachnoid anesthesia may be used when the cervix is completely dilated and when the presenting part is at a level where vaginal delivery can be accomplished.

VI. Labor Pain

A. General considerations. After approximately 266 days of fetal development, a baby is delivered during a physiological process known as labor. Labor pain was essentially a survival mechanism at one time (ie, it warned the mother to decrease activity). The delivery of the fetus is essentially a contest between the forces of expulsion and the forces of resistance. The forces of expulsion involve uterine and abdominal contractions. The forces of resistance include the cervix and pelvis. As is the case with any muscle contraction, labor contractions may be painful. Labor pain may be divided into two distinct types. Nociception mediated through C fiber stimulation is a result of cervical dilatation and cervical effacement. Vaginal and perineal stretching is mediated by A-delta fiber stimulation.

1. In **stage 1**, labor pain is caused by dilatation of the cervix and lower uterine segment. Pain is felt when the uterine contraction pressure exceeds 25 mm Hg or 15 mm Hg above baseline. Afferent nociceptive impulses from the uterus enter the dorsal horn of the spinal cord at T11-12.

    2. In **stage 2**, pain is caused by distention of the lower vagina, vulva, and perineum. Pain is conveyed by sensory pathways that enter the spinal cord through the posterior roots of S2-4.

B. Etiology of labor pain
    1. The etiology is not known but may be caused by decreased oxygen flow to uterine muscle cells, causing ischemic pain, or stretching of the perineum, causing mechanical stimulation of nociceptors or both.
    2. Early labor pain is usually described as dull aching pain, which may be mediated by C fibers.
    3. As labor progresses, sharp pain may be perceived, which may involve A-delta fiber activity, indicating that mechanoreceptors may be involved during stretching of the cervix.

C. Effect of pain
    1. Afferent pain impulses go to the limbic system, which is responsible for the suffering of pain.
    2. When pain is perceived by the brain, the patient's pulse, heart rate, and respiratory rate increase.
    3. Catecholamines are secreted by the adrenal glands during a painful stimulation.
    4. When pain is perceived by the brain, endogenous endorphins are released, but they may not adequately alleviate the pain of labor or may become depleted during the course of labor.

5. Labor pain in some instances can result in decreased oxygen flow to the fetus (uterine artery constriction, increased oxygen consumption).

6. Pain may interfere with the progress of labor.

D. Factors that affect severity of pain

1. In general, older patients experience more intense labor pains.

2. Patients with a history of menstrual difficulties may have decreased pain tolerance and experience more labor pain.

3. The patient who has a minimal understanding of childbirth may have more severe labor pain.

E. Methods of treating labor pain. The fundamental means of decreasing labor pain is to interfere with conduction of afferent or efferent nociceptive impulses, or both.

1. Psychoprophylaxis was introduced in the 1940s by Velvoski. Lamaze introduced this method to the United States after introducing it in France. Patients were taught that labor is painful but that, with maneuvers such as breathing, labor pain can be eliminated or attenuated. The advantage of this method of pain relief is that no medications are administered.

2. Hypnosis modulates afferent pain impulses in the periaqueductal gray matter. Not every patient, however, is able to be adequately hypnotized. The problem with hypnosis is that the hypnotist may not be available for delivery to guide the patient through labor and childbirth.

3. **Transcutaneous electrical nerve stimulator (TENS)** does not eliminate the pain of labor but can attenuate it significantly in some patients. It must be placed properly on the patient to be effective. It may interfere with fetal heart rate monitoring.

4. **Acupuncture.** The needle insertion points using acupuncture to treat labor pain have not been completely worked out. Consequently, pain relief may be inconsistent.

5. **Central nervous system depressants**
   a. **Sedatives (tranquilizers)** are administered to decrease maternal anxiety, which may heighten the experience of pain.
      (1) **Diazepam** has been studied most extensively in the obstetric patient. Diazepam may displace bilirubin from neonatal protein.
      (2) **Midazolam** as well as diazepam can cause maternal amnesia. Both of these drugs in sufficient dosage cause neonatal central nervous system depression.
      (3) **Promethazine and promazine** are effective in decreasing maternal anxiety and cause minimal fetal depression when administered in moderate doses.

      Note: Barbiturates are no longer popular during labor because they may cause fetal depression and can occasionally cause maternal disorientation when a patient experiences severe pain.

b. Opioids, in most instances, are effective for the control of labor pain. Occasionally, parenteral narcotic administration can result in orthostatic hypotension as well as nausea and vomiting. Narcotics can slow the progress of labor if given early during the first stage of labor. Neonatal depression can occur after maternal administration of all opioids; it may be reversed with naloxone.

(1) Butorphanol and nalbuphine are agonist-antagonist opioids that have become increasingly popular for obstetric use. Agonist-antagonist opioids have a respiratory ceiling effect.

(2) Meperidine and morphine are also commonly used in some institutions. Meperidine is one of the most popular drugs currently used in obstetrics. After meperidine administration, if delivery occurs within 2 to 3 hours, the neonate may be depressed.

6. Regional anesthesia

a. Epidural blockade or subarachnoid blockade can be used for the management of pain during the first and second stages of labor. The paracervical block is no longer popular.

b. A subarachnoid block or a pudendal block can be used for the second stage of labor.

SUGGESTED READING

Adams JQ, Alexander AM. Alterations in cardiovascular physiology during labour. *Obstet Gynecol*. 1958; 12:542.

Clark RB. Regional anesthesia. *Obstet Gynecol Annu*. 1984; 13:131.

McKay S, Mahan CS. How worthwhile are membrane stripping and amniotomy? *Contemp Obstet Gynecol*. 1983, Dec. 173.

Melzack R. Labour is still painful after prepared childbirth training. *Can Med Assoc J*. 1981; 125:357.

Scott JR, Rose NB. Effect of psychoprophylaxis (Lamaze preparation) on labor and delivery in primiparas. *N Engl J Med*. 1976; 294:1205.

3

Uteroplacental Circulation and Pharmacodynamics

I. Uterine Blood Flow

At term, uterine blood flow varies from 500 to 700 mL or approximately 10% of the cardiac output.

A. Approximately 80% of uterine blood flow participates in placental exchange.

B. The uterine blood flow is not autoregulated. It is directly dependent upon uterine perfusion pressure and the number and size of the spiral arteries.

C. Factors that decrease uterine blood flow are as follows:

1. Contractions of more than 30 mm Hg
2. Uterine hypertonus
3. Maternal hypotension or hypertension
4. Endogenous or exogenous vasopressors (the uterine vascular bed contains strong alpha-adrenergic receptors)
5. Maternal position (intervillous blood flow has been shown to be lower when the patient is supine versus lateral tilt)

II. Umbilical Blood Flow

A. Approximately 50% of the uterine blood flow is delivered to the placental bed by the umbilical artery.

B. The umbilical blood flow reaches a maximum of 250 mL/minute at term.

III. Placental Transfer

A. General considerations

1. In late pregnancy, the separation between the maternal blood and the fetal endothelium is the syncytiotrophoblast. This placental barrier separates the maternal and fetal blood.

2. The maternal blood is propelled toward the placental basal chorionic plate in fountain-like "spurts" by a pressure head of 70 to 80 torr at the spiral arteries.

3. During contractions, blood flow through the intervillous space is decreased. Consequently, placental exchange continues at a reduced rate.

4. During the stages of gestation, the surface area of the placental membrane increases and its diffusion thickness decreases, thus progressively increasing placental transfer until term. At term, the placental membrane is approximately 3.5 microns in thickness with a total surface area of 11 m² available for exchange. Abruptio placentae, however, decreases the surface area for exchange, and erythroblastosis fetalis, diabetes, and pregnancy-induced hypertension all increase the placental diffusion distance of drugs.

B. Mechanisms of placental transfer. Transfer across the placental barrier is accomplished by different mechanisms, depending on the substance.

1. **Simple diffusion** depends on a concentration gradient and is the principal mode of drug transfer (eg, oxygen, carbon dioxide, small electrolytes).

2. **Active transport** requires a carrier system and energy (eg, amino acids, water-soluble vitamins).

3. **Facilitated diffusion** depends also on a concentration gradient (eg, glucose).

4. **Filtration** depends upon a hydrostatic or pressure gradient (eg, water, some solids).

5. **Pinocytosis:** Transport of substances by enclosure in vesicles formed by the cell membrane that are carried intact to the fetal side of circulation (eg, immunoglobulins, proteins, and other macromolecules).

6. **Breaks in the barrier of the trophoblastic endothelial function** may leak small amounts of plasma and blood cells. As a result, maternal and fetal blood may mix as normal mechanism of placental transfer is bypassed.

C. Rate of placental transfer

1. **Fick's Law of diffusion:**

$$QT = K \cdot A(Cm - Cf)/X$$

where:

- QT = rate of diffusion

- K = diffusion constant of drug
- A = surface area
- Cm = maternal blood concentration
- Cf = fetal blood concentration
- X = thickness of membrane

2. Maternal and pharmacological factors that determine concentration of free drug in uterine artery (Cm) are:
   a. Total drug
   b. Route of administration
   c. Presence of epinephrine in anesthetic solution
   d. Maternal metabolism and excretion
   e. Maternal protein binding
   f. Maternal pH and pKa of a drug

3. Factors that determine concentration of free drug in umbilical artery (Cf) are:
   a. Umbilical venous concentration
   b. Fetal pH
   c. Fetal protein and tissue binding
   d. Non-placental routes of fetal drug elimination—hepatic metabolism and renal excretion. The fetal circulation essentially protects the fetus from the effects of depressant drugs administered to the mother. A large portion of blood passes from the umbilical vein through the fetal liver where it undergoes metabolism. Only one third to two thirds of the maternal blood reaches the inferior vena cava directly through the ductus venosus.
   e. Sluggish, decreased, nonhomogenous blood flow in the intervillous space, which delays equilibration of drug be-

tween the maternal and fetal compartments.

4. Specific drug properties that affect rate of placental transfer
 a. Lipid solubility. Fat-soluble substances like barbiturates and potent inhalational agents pass through the placental membrane very readily.
 b. Molecular weight. As molecular weight increases, substances pass with more difficulty. For example:

MOLECULAR WEIGHT	TRANSFER
<100	Readily
100–600	Slowly
600–1000	Very slowly
>1000	Impermeable

 c. Ionization. The more ionized a substance, the more difficult the transfer of a substance since substances are transferred in the undissociated form.

IV. Anesthetic Considerations
A. General considerations
1. It is imperative that the anesthetist and obstetrician realize that fetal drug effects are frequently difficult to distinguish from maternal events such as umbilical hypoperfusion.
2. Maternal brachial blood pressure readings may not reflect uterine artery perfusion pressure. It is advisable that maternal blood pressure not be allowed to decrease below 100 torr or 20% from preanesthesia values.
3. Administration of a drug just before a

uterine contraction decreases the amount of blood reaching the intervillous space.

4. Rapidly metabolized drugs such as 2-chloroprocaine and succinylcholine are quickly converted to less active metabolites and therefore are considered safer for the fetus as compared to other drugs.

B. Considerations relating to type of anesthesia

1. **Local anesthetics,** especially amides, can depress the fetal myocardium.

2. **General anesthetics** can depress the fetus in a dose-dependent fashion.

3. **Opioids** can depress the neonatal respiratory center.

4. **Thiopental and ketamine** at sufficient fetal plasma levels may also cause neonatal depression. The induction dose of thiopental must be less than 4 mg/kg. The dose of intravenous ketamine should be less than 1 mg/kg.

Note: It is imperative that the anesthetist and obstetrician realize that fetal drug effects are frequently difficult to distinguish from maternal events such as placental hypoperfusion.

SUGGESTED READING

Aherne W, Dunnill MS. Morphometry of the human placenta. *Br Med Bull.* 1966; 22:5.

Gill RW, Trudinger BJ. Garrett WJ et al Fetal umbilical venous flow measured in utero by pulsed Doppler and B-mode ultrasound. *Am J Obstet Gynecol.* 1981; 139:720.

Hagerman DD, Villee CA. Transport functions of the placenta. *Physiol Rev.* 1960; 40:313.

SECTION II

Prepartum Assessment and Management

4

Preanesthetic Assessment and Management

A history and physical examination must be done on all patients before administering any anesthetic. These should be conducted on admission. In doing a system review of the patient's history, an orderly progression must be followed. Once the patient is experiencing pain, she may be unable to give an accurate history and may be difficult to examine.

I. History
   A. Review of systems
   1. Head and neck
      a. Ask about limitations in mouth and jaw range of motion as well as any difficulty with neck extension.
      b. Inquire about any loose teeth, dental appliances, headaches, and seizures.
   2. **Respiratory.** Question the patient regarding smoking, asthma, recent respiratory infection, cough, and dyspnea.
   3. **Cardiovascular**
      a. Inquire about a history of rheumatic fever, palpitations, orthopnea, and

angina (pregnant patients can have ischemic coronary artery disease even though it is rare).

b. Ask the patient if she has been able to lie supine without complications because pregnant patients are prone to caval compression.

4. Endocrine. Ask the patient if she has a history of thyroid disease or diabetes mellitus or any other endocrine history.

5. Hepatic. Inquire about a history of jaundice or hepatitis.

6. Renal. Inquire about a history of kidney or bladder problems.

7. Hematologic. Pregnant patients are essentially hypercoagulable. However, one must elicit a careful history of any bleeding disorders before performing regional anesthesia.

8. Gastrointestinal

a. Ask patients the time of their last food or beverage intake.

b. Inquire about nausea and vomiting, which can occur during pregnancy and which may affect the patient's electrolyte status.

c. A temporary hiatal hernia may be common during pregnancy. Consequently one must inquire about pyrosis (heartburn).

9. Musculoskeletal

a. Pregnant patients can develop significant changes in stance, posture, and gait. Lumbar lordosis may occur during pregnancy. Furthermore, back

pain, muscle pain, and radicular pain can occur during pregnancy. It is important to ask the patient whether or not she has back pain **before** the placement of a regional block.
- **b.** Inquire about any rheumatic disorders during pregnancy.
10. **Genitourinary.** Inquire about a history of herpes simplex virus labialis (HSLV) because epidural morphine may cause a recurrence of HSLV in the postpartum period. The etiology of HSLV is unknown but may be caused by scratching.
11. **Psychiatric.** Ask about a psychiatric history. Local anesthetics at critical levels may exacerbate anxiety attacks.
B. Medications. Ask about any medications that the patient is taking and inquire specifically about beta agonists since they can influence the anesthetic management.
C. Allergies
1. Ask about allergies to medications that the patient may have.
2. Inquire about allergies to suntan lotion (ie, suntan oil may contain para-aminobenzoic acid derivatives [PABA]. Patients allergic to PABA may be allergic to esters).
D. History of previous surgery. A history of previous surgeries, anesthetics, and anesthetic complications must be taken.
E. Family history. Any medical, genetic, or psychiatric history that may affect the patient should be noted.
F. Obstetric history

1. Inquire about any complications with previous pregnancies.
2. Note the mode of delivery of previous pregnancies.
3. Ask the patient if she had an anesthesia for delivery and if there were any complications. Gravidity and parity should be included as well as a history of miscarriage.

G. **Weight gain.** Ask the patient about weight gain. A weight gain of approximately 25 pounds is average. If the patient has significant weight gain before admission, one must think of the possibility of pre-eclampsia. Obesity can increase the incidence of aorto-caval compression.

II. Physical Examination
A. General examination
1. Record the systolic and diastolic blood pressure as well as the pulse and respiratory rates.
2. Make a notation of body build and state of nutrition.
3. Proceed with an orderly progression of the physical examination.

B. Head and neck
1. Note the distance between the thyroid cartilage and mandible, look for loose or missing teeth, and measure jaw range of motion and the jaw opening.
2. Observe the patient for neck extension. Slight physiological enlargement of the thyroid gland is normal.
3. Examine the sclerae for icterus, the pupil

size, and note whether or not the pupils are of equal size bilaterally.

C. Chest. Listen to breath sounds for wheeze, rales, and rhonchi.

D. Cardiovascular. Auscultate the chest for extra heart sounds and murmurs. The intensity of both components of the first heart sound increases during pregnancy. A split first sound may be heard as well as a moderate systolic murmur during pregnancy.

E. Extremities

1. Note deformities or restriction of movement of legs, arms, or back.

2. Palpate the back and spaces between the spinous processes and anticipate difficulty in doing a regional anesthetic.

3. Observe the patient's posture for exaggerated lordosis.

4. Before doing a regional anesthetic, all patients should have a neuromuscular examination testing the patient's reflexes. The following nerves, muscles, and reflexes should be examined and can quickly and easily be done before the administration of regional anesthesia:

a. Peripheral nerves

PERIPH. NERVE	ROOT	MUSCLE	SENSORY DISTRIBUTION	ACTION
Obturator	L2, 3, 4	Adductor longus	Distal medial thigh	Adducts thigh
Femoral	L2, 3, 4	Quadriceps	Distal anterior thigh and posterior calf	Last 10° of knee extension (Continued)

PERIPH. NERVE	ROOT	MUSCLE	SENSORY DISTRIBUTION	ACTION
Sciatic	L4 and S1, 2, 3	Hamstrings	Entire distal leg	Knee flexion
Deep peroneal	L4, S1	Anterior tibial	Web space between 1st and 2nd toes	Dorsiflexes foot

b. Reflexes

1. Patellar reflex: This reflex is mediated through the femoral nerve and L2, 3, 4

2. Achilles reflex: The reflex is mediated through the posterior tibial nerve and Sl-2

III. Review of Patient's Records

If time permits, one should review the patient's previous anesthesia records for information on difficult airway management, difficulty with regional anesthesia, or both. One should be aware of the fact that a previous easy intubation may become difficult in the patient with severe pre-eclampsia.

IV. Subsequent Clinical Assessment

A. Laboratory studies. The appropriate laboratory must be ordered based on the patient's pertinent history and physical examination. Normal laboratory values are presented in the appendix.

B. ASA risk categorization. After the history and physical examination are completed, one should assign a patient classification based on the American Society of Anesthesiologists (ASA) Physical Status Classification as follows:

    I   Normal healthy patient

    II   Mild systemic disease

    III   Severe systemic disease

IV   Severe systemic disease that is a constant threat to life

V   Moribund patient not expected to survive 24 hours with or without the operation

VI   Emergency

C. Anesthetic plan. One must make a notation concerning the type of anesthetic that the anesthetist and patient agreed upon. If the patient is hypovolemic and emergency surgery is indicated, general anesthesia will be necessary. One should also note the fact that all risks of anesthesia were explained to the patient and that the patient understands and accepts these risks.

V. Patient Preparation for Anesthesia and Premedication

A. Insertion of an intravenous line (18 gauge or larger) is essential for all patients before any anesthesia is administered. The purpose of the intravenous line is for hydration and for the administration of drugs and blood should they be needed. Dextrose-containing solutions should not be used for hydration to avoid maternal hypoglycemia and subsequent neonatal hypoglycemia. This is especially important for diabetic patients, who require strict control of blood glucose levels during labor and delivery. Most patients requiring insulin will receive some glucose-containing solution via infusion pump to maintain the blood glucose level within a strict range of 70 to 90 mg/mL. (See Chapter 26 for more detailed information on the management of patients with diabetes mellitus.)

B. **Premedication with an antacid** is essential before induction of general anesthetic to increase the gastric pH to more than 2.5, thus decreasing the incidence of pulmonary aspiration and the risk of pulmonary complications if the patient does aspirate gastric contents. The occurrence and degree of aspiration pneumonitis depends on the pH of aspirated material.

　　1. **Sodium citrate** elevates the gastric pH and has no effect on the volume of gastric acid. Thirty mL of 0.3 molar sodium citrate should be administered before the induction of anesthesia for any cesarean section.

　　2. **Metoclopramide** accelerates gastric emptying and increases lower esophageal sphincter tone. Ten mg intravenously may be given before an emergency cesarean section. Its onset when administered intravenously is 1 to 3 minutes.

　　3. **Cimetidine and ranitidine** are H_2-receptor antagonists. These drugs reduce gastric acidity and gastric volume by blocking gastric histamine H_2 receptors. Ranitidine has a longer duration (6 hours) when compared to cimetidine (4–6 hours). There is an onset time of 60 to 90 minutes when using these drugs. The oral dose of cimetidine is 400 mg followed by 200 mg every 2 hours. The oral dose of ranitidine is 150 mg every 6 hours.

> **Note:** The aspiration of colloidal antacids may produce tissue damage similar to that of acid.

SUGGESTED READING

Ackerman WE, Phero JC. Juneja MM, et al. Panic following 2CP. *Am J Psychiatry.* 1989; 141:940.

Keys A, Fidanza F, Karuonen MJ, et al. Indices of relative weight and obesity. *J Chron Dis.* 1972; 25:329.

Mallampati SR. Clinical signs to predict difficult intubation. *Can Anaesth Soc J.* 1983; 30:316.

Pederson H, Finster M. Anesthetic risk in the pregnant surgical patient. *Anesthesiology.* 1979; 51:439.

Samsoon E, Young R. Difficult tracheal intubation: A retrospective study. *Can Anaesth Soc J.* 1987; 42:487.

5

Prepartum Fetal Assessment

Patients who require antepartum fetal assessment are usually patients with hypertension, kidney disease, diabetes, pre-eclampsia, and intrauterine growth retardation. Fetal monitoring is employed for antepartum assessment of the fetus. (Refer to Chapter 13, Fetal Monitoring.)

I. Non-Stress Test
   Is useful for determining fetal well-being. It is obtained with the parturient in the semi-Fowler's position for at least 20 minutes.
   A. Reactive test. By the Evertson criteria, reactivity consists of an acceleration of 15 beats/minute with a duration of at least 15 seconds, which occurs twice in 20 minutes, with fetal movement.
   B. Nonreactive test. Absence of movements with accelerations for 40 minutes.
   C. Advantages: Sensitive test. Inexpensive.
   D. Disadvantages: False-positive rate of 20 to 80%.

II. Contraction Stress Test
   May be used as a follow-up to the non-stress

test. Oxytocin is administered intravenously and the dose is increased every 15 to 20 minutes until three contractions are noted within a 10-minute period.

A. Positive test. Deceleration noted with 50% of the contractions.

B. Negative test. No deceleration noted with three contractions in 10 minutes.

C. Equivocal. Late decelerations noted but not recurrent.

D. Advantages: Most sensitive antepartum test.

E. Disadvantages: Time consuming. Requires intravenous administration of a medication.

III. Real-Time Ultrasonography

Identifies congenital anomalies when they are present, as well as intrauterine growth retardation.

A. Advantages: Can diagnose congenital malformations, amniotic fluid volume, and placenta previa.

B. Disadvantages: No major disadvantages related to ultrasonography.

IV. Amniocentesis

Amniocentesis is the placement of a needle through the uterus, into the amniotic sac, from which amniotic fluid is aspirated.

A. Advantages: The lecithin sphingomyelin (L/S) ratio can be determined. An L/S ratio of 2.0 is an indicator of lung maturity. Chromosome abnormalities and fetal sex can be determined by amniocentesis. Alpha fetoprotein may also be measured, which may be elevated if fetal anomalies or distress exist.

B. Disadvantages: Amnionitis, peritonitis, and hemorrhage.

V. Estriol Level

Plasma estriol levels increase throughout gestation. In the maternal-fetal-placental unit, estriol is formed from fetal dehydroepiandrosterone sulfate. A 50% decrease from a previous value or a 30% decrease from its mean value of three previous levels should be reason for a contraction stress test.

A. Advantages: How levels are associated with a high evidence of congenital anomalies, and intrauterine death.

B. Disadvantages: Corticosteroids and ampicillin ingested by the patient may yield low estriol levels.

SUGGESTED READING

Boehm FH, Srisupundit S, Ishii T et al. Lecithin-sphingomyelin ratio and a rapid test for surfactant in amniotic fluid. A comparison. *Obstet Gynecol.* 1973; 41:829.

Magendantz HG, Ryan KJ. Isolation of an estriol precursor, 16 alpha-hydroxy-dehydroepiandrosterone from human umbilical sera. *J Clin Endocrinol Metab.* 1964; 28:1155.

Milunsky A. Prenatal detection of neural tube defects. VI. Experience with 20,000 pregnancies. *JAMA.* 1980; 244:2731.

Rochard F, Schifrin BS. Goupii F et al. Non-stressed fetal heart rate monitoring in the antepartum period. *Am J Obstet Gynecol.* 1976; 126:699.

Whitfield CR. The diagnostic value of amniocentesis. *Clin Obstet Gynecol.* 1974; 1:67.

SECTION III

Perinatal Pharmacology

6

Drugs Commonly Used in Obstetrics

I. Narcotics

Narcotics are the naturally occurring alkaloids of opium. The term **opioids** describes narcotics as well as the synthetic and semisynthetic derivatives. Opioids may stimulate mu or kappa opioid receptors, which results in analgesia. The mu receptor opioids most commonly used for labor analgesia are morphine, meperidine, and fentanyl. Mu receptor-stimulating opioids are referred to as agonists. Another classification of opioids are the mixed agonist-antagonist opioids. The two commonly used in labor include butorphanol and nalbuphine. These opioids act on both mu and kappa receptors or stimulate both mu and kappa receptors. Mixed agonist-antagonist opioids exhibit less respiratory depression at therapeutic doses.

A. Use in obstetrics. Narcotics may be used for analgesia during the first stage of labor.

B. Contraindications. Contraindications to opioids include allergies to a particular drug. One should not give an agonist-antagonist opioid to a patient who is a narcotic abuser.

C. Toxicity and side effects. Narcotics in general can exhibit the following side effects:
   1. Decreased gastric motility and lower esophageal sphincter tone.
   2. Emetic effects.
   3. Can cause neonatal depression.
D. Specific narcotic agents
   1. Agonist opioids
      a. Meperidine is the most popular narcotic used currently by obstetricians in North America.
         (1) Dosage: 50 to 100 mg IM or 25 to 50 mg IV
         (2) Peak effect: 40 to 50 minutes after intramuscular injection; 5 to 10 minutes after IV injection
         (3) Duration of action: approximately 3 hours
      b. Morphine. Morphine may be used for analgesia during labor and is usually administered intramuscularly.
         (1) Dosage: 5 to 10 mg IM
         (2) Peak effect: 1 to 2 hours after intramuscular injection
         (3) Duration of action: 4 to 6 hours
      c. Fentanyl is not commonly used for analgesia other than epidurally. It may be given (50 μg intravenously) to provide rapid relief to a patient who is unable to cooperate during placement of an epidural needle.
   2. Mixed agonist-antagonist opioids
      a. Butorphanol
         (1) Dosage: 2 mg IM; 0.5 to 1 mg IV
         (2) Peak effect: similar to morphine

       (3) Duration of action: approximately 4 hours

   b. Nalbuphine. The dosage, peak effect, and duration of action of nalbuphine are similar to morphine (see **1.b** above).

II. Tocolytic Agents

Tocolytic agents are drugs used to slow or stop labor. Tocolytic agents include beta-2 agonists, magnesium sulfate, and calcium channel blockers. Beta-adrenergic receptors can be divided into two groups: beta-1 activity is manifest as an increase in heart rate and contractility. Beta-2 receptor activity causes bronchodilation, vasodilation, and uterine relaxation. Calcium channel blockers are currently investigational.

A. Beta agonists. Ritodrine, isoxsuprine, and terbutaline all are selective beta-2 agonists.

B. Use in obstetrics. Beta-2 adrenergic agonists produce a more rapid onset of tocolysis when compared to magnesium sulfate. Beta-2 agonists are used in preference to magnesium sulfate in emergent situations.

C. Contraindications to beta agonists as tocolytic agents are:

   1. Heart disease

   2. Hyperthyroidism

   3. Cerebral ischemia

   4. Hypovolemia

   5. Maternal infection

D. Toxicity and side effects

   1. Tachycardia

   2. Decreased systemic vascular resistance

   3. Arrhythmias

    4. Hypokalemia

    5. Pulmonary edema (often associated with prehydration; may be related to increased pulmonary capillary permeability)

E. Specific beta agonist agents

    1. Ritodrine (Yotopar) is the only beta agonist that is FDA approved for use as a tocolytic agent.

        a. Dosage: 50 to 100 μg by IV infusion. The dose can be increased by 50 Mcg for a maximum dose of 350 mg/minute. After contractions stop, 10 to 20 mg q4—6h PO for a maximum dose of 120 mg.

        b. Onset: Less than 10 minutes IV; 30 to 60 minutes PO.

        c. Duration of action: IV 2 to 2.5 hours; PO 12 hours.

    2. Isoxsuprine and terbutaline are beta agonists pending FDA approval for use as tocolytic agents. Ritodrine and terbutaline are both more beta-2 specific than isoxsuprine.

F. Magnesium sulfate. Magnesium sulfate exhibits a mild antihypertensive effect. Diminishes central nervous system excitability and interferes with the release of acetylcholine at the neuromuscular junction.

    1. Dosage: 4 g IV over 15 minutes, followed by 1 g/hour.

    2. Onset: IV; immediate.

    3. Duration: 30 minutes.

    4. Side effects: Depends on plasma level. Therapeutic level is 4 to 8 mEq/L. Higher levels may result in side effects ranging from loss of deep tendon reflexes 10 mEq/L—cardiac arrest (30 mEq/L).

III. Oxytocic Agents

Oxytocic agents stimulate the uterus to contract. Oxytocin may be used to stimulate labor. If uterine atony exists, however, methylergonovine or prostaglandin-2 alpha may be used.

A. Use in obstetrics. As mentioned, oxytocic agents.

B. Contraindications.

C. Specific oxytocic drugs

1. **Synthetic oxytocin** is a hormone that stimulates uterine contractions. The uterus reaches its maximum sensitivity to oxytocin at 34 to 36 weeks. Its plasma half-life is 2 to 9 minutes when administered intravenously. It is metabolized by plasma and placental oxytocinase.

   a. **Dosage:** 20 to 40 units/1000 mg Ringer's lactate given by continuous IV infusion up to 200 mL/hour.

   b. **Onset:** The onset of oxytocin is less than one minute

   c. **Duration of action:** 2 to 3 minutes

   d. **Toxicity and side effects:**

      (1) Because there is a tremendous variation in sensitivity to oxytocin, overstimulation of the uterus may occur and result in uterine tetany and rupture as well as fetal distress and asphyxia.

      (2) Oxytocin can have a antidiuretic hormonal (AD) effect. Water intoxication can occur with large

amounts of electrolyte-free solution.

(3) Following oxytocin administration, the mean arterial pressure can decrease 30%; the total peripheral resistance can decrease 50%; the pulse can increase 30%; and the cardiac output can increase 50%. These events can result in tachycardia or hypotension. Hypotension is less likely to occur with a dilute solution.

2. **Methylergonovine maleate (Methergine)** has been used successfully to treat uterine atony unresponsive to oxytocin. Methergine is an ergot alkaloid that produces uterine contractions.

   a. **Dosage:** 0.2 mg IM. It should **not** be given intravenously in hypertensive patients, since methergine can cause more severe hypertension. Therefore, this drug should be used judiciously in hypertensive patients.

   b. **Onset:** 2 to 5 minutes following intramuscular injection.

   c. **Duration of action:** 3 to 4 hours.

   d. **Side effects:**
      (1) Hypertension
      (2) May possibly cause coronary artery spasm

3. **Prostaglandin F$_2$ alpha** is a hormone that produces uterine contractions. It exerts its pharmacological action through enhancement of calcium transport through the uterine muscle cell membrane.

    a. Dosage: 1 mg intramyometrially
    b. Peak effect: 1 to 3 minutes
    c. Duration of action: 90 minutes
    d. Side effects:
        (1) Nausea or emesis
        (2) Vomiting
        (3) Fever

SUGGESTED READING

Fishburne TI. Systemic analgesia during labor. *Clin Perinatol.* 1982; 9:33.

Hodgkinson R, Husain FJ. The duration of effect of maternally administered meperidine on neonatal neurobehavior. *Anesthesiology.* 1982; 56:51.

Merkatz IR, Peter JB, Barden TP. Ritodrine hydrochloride: A betamimetic agent for use in preterm labor. II. Evidence of efficacy. *Obstet Gynecol.* 1980; 56:7.

Stubblefield PG, Heyl PS. Treatment of premature labor with subcutaneous terbutaline. *Obstet Gynecol.* 1982; 59:457.

7

Epidural and Subarachnoid Opioids

I. General

A. The use of intraspinal opioids in labor has become increasingly popular. Furthermore, intraspinal opioids are also popular for postoperative pain.

B. Preservative-free morphine is currently the only FDA-approved narcotic for epidural use. Reports of epidural fentanyl and other epidural opioids, however, are becoming prevalent in the obstetric anesthesia literature.

C. Intraspinal morphine, which has a relatively low lipid solubility, may exhibit an increased cephalad spread when compared to epidural fentanyl, which has a much higher lipid solubility.

D. Epidural fentanyl is rapidly removed from the CSF in contrast to epidural morphine, which is removed much slower from the CNS.

E. One of the positive attributes of epidural opioids during labor is that less concentration of local anesthetic is used, thus preserving motor functions and decreasing the total mass of local anesthetic that both the mother and fetus are exposed to.

F. Epidural narcotics can be given in a bolus (ie, 50 μg fentanyl with 0.25% bupivacaine) or in a continuous infusion (ie, 1 μg/mL with 0.125% bupivacaine).

G. Side effects:

   1. Pruritus is the most common side effect. Pruritus is worse in the parturient following epidural morphine administration (incidence: 50 to 70%).

   2. Respiratory depression is a rare complication but may nevertheless occur (incidence: 0.09% epidural; 0.36% intrathecal).

   3. Nausea or emesis, or both, can occur following epidural opioid administration (incidence: 25% epidural narcotics; 50% intrathecal narcotics).

   4. Urinary retention has also been shown to occur (incidence: 22 to 50%).

   5. Respiratory depression can occur if there is rapid vascular absorption or if another CNS depressant drug is used systemically.

II. Neonatal Effects

A. There have been no neonatal side effects reported nor any significant differences noted in neonatal Apgar scores following epidural morphine administration in labor.

B. To date, no neonatal side effects have been reported following epidural fentanyl or intrathecal fentanyl.

C. A sinusoidal fetal heart tracing has been reported following butorphanol administration (3 mg).

D. It may not be advisable to administer epidural narcotics to any patient whose fetus shows any signs of distress until further studies are done.

III. Neurotoxicity

A. Neither morphine, buprenorphine, meperidine, fentanyl, nor butorphanol without preservatives has been found to be neurotoxic.

B. Reversal

   1. The standard for instant reversal of opioid side effects is naloxone.

   2. Naloxone has been shown not to reverse epidural analgesia following the administration of epidural narcotics. The dose is 5 µg/kg.

   3. Naltrexone has a longer duration of action than naloxone. It may be administered PO (5 to 6 mg diluted in a cola drink).

IV. Anesthetic Considerations

A. Epidural narcotics alone, other than sufentanil, are not effective during labor. The reason may be that alpha-delta fibers are not adequately blocked by narcotics alone.

B. Fentanyl has been shown to potentiate the effects of bupivacaine.

C. Sherman et al have demonstrated that 0.25% bupivacaine with 1 µg/mL fentanyl provided superior analgesia when followed after 20 minutes with a continuous epidural infusion of 0.125% bupivacaine with 2.5 µg/mL of fentanyl at 10 mL/hour.

D. Cohen et al, however, did not show the combination of 50 to 100 µg of fentanyl added to 0.25% bupivacaine to increase effectiveness. These authors, however, did not report the effects of a continuous infusion.

E. Pruritus is common following administration of epidural fentanyl or morphine. Furthermore, recurrence of herpes simplex virus labialis (HSVL) can be increased in the parturient who received epidural morphine, which may be caused by scratching.

F. It is controversial whether or not any patient who has a history of HSVL may be a candidate for epidural opioids as scratching may cause reactivation.

G. Intrathecal morphine, 0.25 mg, administered in combination with 25 μg of fentanyl has been shown to be effective for the first stage of labor.

V. Use of Epidural Opioids for Postcesarean Section Pain

A. Epidural morphine is the only opioid currently approved for epidural use. For postoperative pain, 5 mg has been shown to be effective. Because morphine has relatively low lipid solubility, its onset may take from 30 to 60 minutes. Consequently, one may administer epidural morphine soon after delivery.

B. The addition of 0.125% bupivacaine has not been shown to affect the quality or duration of analgesia provided by epidural morphine. The benefit of giving epidural morphine for postcesarean section pain is that epidural administration produces analgesia for a much longer time.

C. Serum levels after epidural administration of opioids are similar to those occurring after the same dose is given intramuscularly. Adverse side effects following the epidural use of opioids for pain include nausea, emesis, pruritus, urinary retention, and respiratory depression.

D. The incidence of pruritus following epidural administration of morphine is dose dependent. The side effects of epidural opioids may be attenuated with naloxone.

E. There is an increased incidence of HSVL following epidural morphine administration.

VI. Other Drugs

A. Epidural fentanyl, meperidine, hydromorphone, buprenorphine, and butorphanol were reported to be effective in management of postcesarean section pain.

B. Of these epidural opioids, buprenorphine provided the longest duration of analgesia with less pruritus than fentanyl and less sedation than butorphanol when administered epidurally for the management of postoperative cesarean section pain.

C. Sufentanil, 30 μg, has been shown to provide adequate postoperative analgesia with minimal narcotic-induced side effects.

D. Hydromorphone, 1 mg with 9 mL of saline, has also been shown to provide adequate postoperative analgesia.

E. A total volume (opioid and saline) of 10 mL has been shown to be a critical value for providing analgesia.

F. The use of 2-chloroprocaine with epidural morphine or fentanyl, or both, may decrease the efficacy of both of these opioids.

VII. Intrathecal Opioids

A. Morphine provides analgesia within 30 minutes and fentanyl within 5 minutes.

B. Before cesarean section, 0.2 to 0.5 mg of morphine may be administered for postoperative analgesia.

SUGGESTED READING

Ackerman WE, Juneja MM, Colclough G. A comparison of epidural fentanyl, buprenorphine, and butorphanol for the management of post cesarean section pain. *Anesthesiology*. 1988; 69:A401.

Chestnut DH, Choi WW, Isbell TJ. Epidural hydromorphone for post cesarean analgesia. *Obstet Gynecol*. 1986; 68:65.

Cohen SE, Tan S, White PF. Sufentanil analgesia following cesarean section. Epidural versus intravenous administration. *Anesthesiology*. 1988; 68:129.

Douglas MJ, McMorland GH, Janzen JA. Influence of bupivacaine as an adjuvant to epidural morphine for analgesia after cesarean section. *Anesth Analg*. 1985; 67:1138.

Gieraerts R, Navalgund A, Vaes L, et al. Increased incidence of morphine after cesarean section. *Anesth Analg*. 1987; 66:1321.

Gieraerts R, Navalgund A, Vaes L, et al. Increased incidence of itching and herpes simplex in patients given epidural morphine after cesarean section. *Anesth Analg*. 1987; 66:1321.

Hughes S, Rosen MA, Shnider SM, et al. Maternal and neonatal effects of epidural morphine for labor and delivery. *Anesth Analg*. 1984; 63:319.

Justins DM, Francis D, Houlton PG. A controlled trial of extradural fentanyl in labour. *Br J Anesth*. 1983; 54:409.

Kotelko DM, Thigpen JW, Shnider SM, et al. Postoperative

epidural morphine analgesia after various local anesthetics. *Anesthesiology*. 1983; 59:A413.

Leighton BL, DeSimore CA, Norris MC, et al. Intrathecal narcotics for labor revisited: The combination of fentanyl and morphine intrathecally provides rapid onset of profound prolonged analgesia. *Anesth Analg*. 1989; 69:122.

Rosen MA, Hughes SC, Shnider SM, et al. Epidural morphine for the relief of postoperative pain after cesarean delivery. *Anesth Analg*. 1983; 62:666.

Sherman JH, Thompson RA, Goldstern MT, et al. Combined continuous epidural fentanyl and bupivacaine in labor: A randomized study. *Anesthesiology*. 1985; 63:A450.

8

Local Anesthetic Considerations

Local anesthetics inhibit nociceptive impulses during the first and second stages of labor. There are two groups of local anesthetics: amino esters and amino amides. They differ pharmacologically in that esters have an ester linkage in the molecule, while amides have an amide linkage in their molecular structure. Amide local anesthetics are essentially metabolized by the liver, while esters are metabolized by plasma pseudocholinesterase. The molecular weights of the local anesthetics used in obstetric anesthesia vary between 200 and 300. The local anesthetics are furthermore lipophilic and can easily cross the placenta. Placental transfer is also influenced by the pKa of the local anesthetics as well as by the pH of the maternal and fetal blood. Ester local anesthetics are metabolized rapidly by maternal plasma pseudocholinesterase and, in general, do not accumulate in the fetus.

I. Use in Obstetric Anesthesia
Both amides and esters are used for subarachnoid and epidural block for labor, vaginal delivery, and cesarean section.

II. Contraindications
Allergy to a specific local anesthetic.

III. Toxicity and Side Effects
A. Maternal. The central nervous system, respiratory system, and cardiovascular system, may all be adversely affected by local anesthetics.

1. **Central nervous system** side effects include:
   a. Numbness of the tongue
   b. Lightheadedness or dizziness
   c. Disorientation
   d. Convulsions
2. **Respiratory system.** An initial increase or decrease in respiratory rate may be noted, which may progress to apnea and respiratory arrest.
3. **Cardiovascular system.** Cardiac conduction and contractility can be decreased, which may progress to asystole. With some agents, especially bupivacaine, cardiac arrhythmias and cardiac arrest may occur.

B. Fetal. At present, abnormal fetal neurobehavioral scores following administration of local anesthetics for epidural block are controversial.

IV. Specific Drugs
See Chapter 11, Regional Anesthetic Considerations, for specific doses used in subarachnoid block and epidural block.

A. Esters. The commonly used ester agents are 2-chloroprocaine and tetracaine.

1. **2-Chloroprocaine** has the shortest plasma life of all anesthetics. The rate of hydrolysis is 4.7 μmol/mL/hour. It under-

goes rapid esterification and therefore has minimal cumulative fetal toxicity.

a. Concentration

(1) 2% for labor (and vaginal delivery)

(2) 3% for cesarean section

b. Onset of effect: 4 to 6 minutes

c. Duration of action: Short duration of action (30 to 60 minutes) requiring frequent top-up doses.

d. Special indications. Has been recommended for labor with fetal distress.

e. pKa: 8.7

f. Protein binding: Metabolized rapidly by plasma pseudocholinesterase.

g. Umbilical vein/maternal vein ratio: Unknown. Chloroprocaine reaches the fetus in minute amounts.

h. Advantages: Rapid onset. Rapid metabolism decreases the incidence of ion trapping.

i. Disadvantages: Short duration of action. Question of neurological sequelae if administered in subarachnoid space.

j. Specific toxicities and side effects. There have been reports of prolonged sensory and motor deficits following administration of a large volume into the subarachnoid space. The specific volume necessary to result in neurological damage is currently unknown.

2. Tetracaine. Tetracaine is administered in the subarachnoid space for the second stage of labor and for anesthesia for cesarean section.

a. Concentration: 1%

   b. Onset of effect: 5 to 10 minutes
   c. Duration of action: 60 to 180 minutes
   d. Special indications: None
   e. pKa: 8.3
   f. Protein binding: 75%
   g. Umbilical vein/maternal vein ratio: Unknown
   h. Advantages: Relatively long duration
   i. Disadvantages: Relatively high toxicity
   j. Specific toxicities and side effect: No different than other local anesthetics.
 B. Amide agents. Lidocaine and bupivacaine are the most commonly used of the various amide agents.
  1. Lidocaine
   a. Concentration: 1, 1.5, 2, and 5% solutions. The 5% concentration is used for subarachnoid anesthesia
   b. Onset of effect: 5 to 15 minutes
   c. Duration: 60 to 75 minutes
   d. Special indication: None
   e. pKa: 7.9
   f. Protein binding: 64%
   g. Umbilical vein/maternal vein ratio: 0.6
   h. Advantages: Fast onset
   i. Disadvantages: Tachyphylaxis may occur during epidural administration
   j. Specific toxicities and side effects: Similar to other local anesthetics. Premature fetal sheep have shown myocardial depression associated with significant plasma lidocaine levels following epidural administration.

2. Bupivacaine
   a. Concentration: 0.25, 0.5, and 0.75% should not be used for epidural anesthesia in pregnant patients
   b. Onset of effect: 10 to 20 minutes
   c. Duration: 90 to 120 minutes
   d. Specific indications: None
   e. pKa: 8.1
   f. Protein binding: 95%
   g. Umbilical vein/maternal vein ratio: 0.4
   h. Advantages: Long duration of action
   i. Disadvantages: Myocardial toxicity
   j. Specific toxicities and side effects: Cardiac toxicity may be noted in patients that are hypoxic and acidotic
3. Etidocaine
   a. Concentration: 1 and 1.5%
   b. Onset of effect: 5 to 15 minutes
   c. Duration: 90–180 minutes
   d. Special indications: Usually used for cesarean sections when one wants profound muscle relaxation
   e. pKa: 7.7
   f. Protein binding: 94%
   g. Umbilical vein/maternal vein ratio: 0.30
   h. Advantages: Fast onset. Good muscle relaxation for cesarean section
   i. Disadvantages: Not useful for labor because of profound muscle relaxation
   j. Specific toxicities and side effects: Potential for cardiac toxicity may be similar to bupivacaine
4. Prilocaine: It is not used in obstetric an-

esthesia because fetal plasma levels may exceed maternal levels, and because maternal and fetal methemoglobinemia may occur.

5. **Mepivacaine:** It is not used in obstetric anesthesia because it can have a long neonatal half-life (9 hours) and because mepivacaine has been associated with neonatal neurobehavioral changes.

C. **Use of epinephrine with local anesthetics.** Epinephrine added to local anesthetics prolongs the duration of spinal anesthetics. Epinephrine reduces lidocaine maternal plasma levels, but has minimal effect on bupivacaine and etidocaine levels. Epinephrine may prolong the effects of epidural lidocaine.

1. **Indications:** To prolong spinal anesthesia.

2. **Relative contraindications:** Hypertension, arrhythmias, myocardial ischemia.

D. **Top-up doses.** A top-up dose is a reinjection of a local anesthetic through an existing epidural catheter. The volume of local anesthetic for top-up dose is essentially a test dose and must be given slowly; and signs of subarachnoid and intravascular injection must be monitored. See Chapter 11, Regional Anesthetic Considerations, for specific top-up doses in subarachnoid and epidural block.

SUGGESTED READING

Abboud TH, Khoo SS, Miller Q, et al. Maternal, fetal and neonatal responses after epidural anesthesia with bupivacaine, 2-chloroprocaine or lidocaine. *Anesth Analg*. 1982; 61:638.

Bromage PR, Pettugrew RT, Crowell DE. Tachyphylaxis in epidural analgesia. I. Augmentation and decay of local anesthesia. *J Clin Pharmacol*. 1969; 9:30.

deJong RH, Ronfeld RA, deRosa RA, et al. Cardiovascular effects of convulsant and supraconvulsant doses of amide local anesthetics. *Anesth Analg*. 1982; 61:3.

Kasten GW, Martin ST. Successful resuscitation after massive intravenous bupivacaine overdose in anesthetized dogs. *Anesthesiology*. 1985; 64:491.

Scanlon JW, Ostheimer GW, Lurie AO, et al. Neurobehavioral response and drug concentrations in newborns after maternal epidural anesthesia with bupivacaine. *Anesthesiology*. 1976; 45:400.

Scott DB. Toxicity caused by local anesthetic drugs. *Br J Anaesth*. 1981; 53:553.

9

Inhalation Agents

Inhalational analgesia is the administration of inhalational anesthetics in concentrations less than that required for surgical anesthesia during the first and second stages of labor. The mother should remain awake throughout this technique and should maintain protective laryngeal reflexes.

I. Techniques of Inhalational Analgesia
   A. May be administered intermittently (during contractions) or continuously.
   B. If administered intermittently, it should be administered approximately 30 seconds before the onset of a contraction to provide adequate analgesia for the contraction.
   C. The concentration should be adjusted to a patient's response.
   D. If a patient becomes progressively drowsy, the concentration should be decreased.
   E. Continuous inhalational analgesia offers a continuous level of analgesia.

II. Advantages
   A. Rapid reversibility.
   B. Patient remains conscious.

C. No adverse effects on mother or baby.
III. Disadvantages
    A. If the patient becomes obtunded, one must worry about the patient's protective airway reflexes.
    B. Environmental pollution
IV. Apparatus
    A. Anesthetic machine
    B. Flow-over vaporizer
V. Agents
    A. Nitrous oxide: One may use a 50% mixture with oxygen.
        1. Advantage: Safe.
        2. Disadvantage: May cause restlessness.
    B. Methoxyflurane: A 0.3 to 0.5% concentration has been shown to be efficacious.
        1. Advantage: Does not cause restlessness.
        2. Disadvantage: Environmental pollution. Potential for nephrotoxicity from high levels of metabolites.
    C. Halothane: Its use as an analgesic is controversial because of the potential for uterine relaxation.
    D. Isoflurane: Has not been extensively studied for obstetric use.
    E. Enflurane: Ethrane is a potent analgesic when administered at subanesthetic concentrations.
        1. Advantage: Excellent analgesic and is rapidly eliminated by the neonate.
        2. Disadvantage: Possible potential for seizure activity if patient hyperventilates.
VI. General Considerations
    A. Maternal safety. One must always observe

for loss of consciousness and the loss of protective laryngeal reflexes.

B. 30 mL of a non-particulate antacid should be administered to all patients having inhalational analgesia.

C. The anesthetist must remain in verbal contact with the patient.

D. The blood pressure should be checked every 5 minutes.

E. Prolonged administration may result in neonatal depression.

SUGGESTED READING

Clark RB, Beard AG, Thompson DS, et al. Maternal and neonatal plasma inorganic fluoride levels after methoxyflurane analgesia for labor and delivery. *Anesthesiology.* 1976; 45:89.

McGuinness C, Rosen M. Enflurane as an analgesic in labour. *Anaesthesia.* 1984; 39:27.

Rosen M, Mushin WW, Jones PL, et al. Field trial of methoxyflurane, nitrous oxide and trichloroethylene as obstetric analgesics. *Br Med J.* 1969; 3:263.

Waud BE, Waud DR. Calculated kinetics of distribution of nitrous oxide and methoxyflurane during intermittent administration in obstetrics. *Anesthesiology.* 1970; 32:306.

Wilson RD, Priano LL, Allen CR, et al. Demand analgesia and anesthesia in obstetrics. *South Med J.* 1972; 65:556.

10

Drug Interactions

The use of some drugs used in the practice of obstetrics may alter or affect drugs used in the practice of obstetric anesthetic considerations.

I. Antacids
  A. Cimetidine
   1. Mechanism of action: Inhibits histamine (H_2) at parietal cell receptor sites. Decreases gastric acid secretion.
   2. Side effects: Mental confusion on occasion or dizziness. Bradycardia may be noted on occasion.
   3. Interactions: Inhibition of hepatic microsomal enzyme metabolism of amide local anesthetics, benzodiazepines, and propranolol.
  B. Ranitidine
   1. Mechanism of action: Same as cimetidine.
   2. Side effects: Similar to cimetidine.
   3. Interactions: Less of an effect on hepatic microsomal enzymes when compared to cimetidine.

II. Oxytocics
A. Oxytocin
1. **Mechanism of action:** Selective stimulator of uterine and mammary gland smooth muscle.
2. **Side effects:** Water intoxication from antidiuretic effects, hypotension, tachycardia.
3. **Interactions:** Delayed induction possible following thiopental administration. Hypertension following oxytocin administration in patient who received methoxamine administered prophylactically. Ephedrine may also result in hypertension when administered with oxytocin.

B. Methylergonovine maleate
1. **Mechanism of action:** Uterine contraction is a result of direct stimulation.
2. **Side effects:** Headache, dizziness, hypertension, heart palpitations.
3. **Interactions:** With local anesthetics, dopamine, and intravenous oxytocin. Vasoconstriction can occur following administration, resulting in severe hypertension.
4. **Precaution:** Administer intramuscularly. Avoid in pre-eclamptic patients and in patients with cardiac disease where increases in the systemic vascular resistance may be detrimental (ie, mitral or aortic insufficiency).

III. Tocolytics
A. Magnesium sulfate
1. **Mechanism of action:** Decreases acetylcholine release at nerve ending.

2. Side effects: Drowsiness, decreased reflexes, flaccid paralysis, hypotension.

3. Interactions: Potentiates both depolarizing and non-depolarizing muscle relaxants. For this reason, pretreatment with curare is not recommended for general anesthesia in patients receiving magnesium sulfate because total paralysis could occur. Non-depolarizing muscle relaxants should be titrated using a nerve stimulator. Because of the ability of magnesium sulfate to decrease a parturient's blood pressure, one must closely monitor the blood pressure during the administration of both regional and general anesthesia.

B. Ritodrine hydrochloride

1. Mechanism of action: Stimulates beta-2-adrenergic receptors in uterine smooth muscle, which inhibits uterine muscle contractility.

2. Side effects: Anxiety, headaches, palpitations, hypokalemia, tachycardia, palpitations, pulmonary edema, increase in cardiac output, hyperglycemia.

3. Interactions: When used in combination with steroids, pulmonary edema may occur. Beta blockers may inhibit the action of ritodrine. Halothane use may result in dysrhythmias. May cause severe hypertension when administered with sympathomimetics.

C. Terbutaline (Not FDA approved at present.)

1. Mechanism of action: Similar to ritodrine.

2. Side effects: Similar to ritodrine.
3. Interactions: Similar to ritodrine.

SUGGESTED READING

Barden TP, Peter JB, Merkatz IR, et al. Ritodrine hydrochloride: Betamimetic agent for use in preterm labor. *Obstet Gynecol*. 1980; 56:1.

Caritis SN, Edelstone DI, Mueller-Heubach E. Pharmacologic inhibition of preterm labor. *Am J Obstet Gynecol*. 1979; 133:557.

Devore JS, Asrani R. Magnesium sulfate prevents succinylcholine-induced fasciculation in toxemic parturients. *Anesthesiology*. 1980; 52:76.

Morris R, Giesecke AH. Of magnesium, muscle relaxants, toxemic parturients and cats. *Anesth Analg*. 1968; 147:689.

Weis FR, Markello R, Benjamen MO. Cardiovascular effects of oxytocin. *Obstet Gynecol*. 1975; A6:211.

SECTION IV

Techniques of Obstetric Anesthesia

11

Types of Obstetric Regional Anesthesia

In the practice of obstetric anesthesia, regional anesthesia is popular with the parturient because the patient may remain awake and can immediately interact with her baby without being overly sedated with narcotics or tranquilizers. Epidural anesthesia is becoming increasingly popular for labor and delivery, as well as for cesarean section. Epidural narcotics may be administered for postoperative pain control. Spinal anesthesia is popular for the second stage of labor, and in some centers, is preferred by some anesthetists over lumbar epidural anesthesia for cesarean section.

I. Epidural Anesthesia
A. Advantages:
1. Continuous analgesia during labor.
2. Slow onset when compared to spinal anesthesia and, therefore, a decreased incidence of hypotension, decreased incidence of postdural puncture head-

ache, and postcesarean or postepi-
siotomy pain.

3. Management may be accomplished
through use of an epidural catheter post-
delivery.

B. Disadvantages:

1. Slower onset compared to spinal anesthesia.

2. Technically more difficult to perform than
spinal anesthesia.

3. On occasion, may be difficult to provide
adequate anesthesia for cesarean section.

C. Contraindications: Hemorrhage, coagulopathies, septicemia, and infection over the
epidural needle puncture site.

II. Caudal Block

A caudal block may occasionally be used in instances where a double catheter technique is
used. The advantage of this technique is that
T_{10}-L_1 can be selectively anesthetized for the
first stage of labor and the sacral fibers can be
anesthetized. It may also be used to establish
perineal anesthesia in instances where one is
unable to establish perineal anesthesia by the
lumbar epidural route.

A. Advantages: Providing perineal anesthesia
when a controlled vaginal delivery is desirable.

B. Disadvantages: The volume of local anesthetic needed to establish anesthesia may
be greater than that for lumbar epidural anesthesia and risk of infection exists.

C. Contraindications: Same as for epidural anesthesia.

III. Spinal Anesthesia

Spinal anesthesia is effective for the second stage of delivery and for cesarean section. Continuous spinal anesthesia is currently investigational.

A. Advantages:
1. Quick onset.
2. Greater reliability.

B. Disadvantages:
1. Hypotension may occur with a greater incidence with spinal anesthesia than with epidural anesthesia.
2. The incidence of postdural puncture headaches is increased following spinal anesthesia.

C. Contraindications: Hypovolemia, meningitis, infection at puncture site, bleeding problems.

IV. Pudendal Block

A pudendal block provides anesthesia for the second stage of labor. It also provides anesthesia for forceps delivery.

A. Advantages:
1. Ease of administration.
2. Minimal maternal hypotension.

B. Disadvantages:
1. Not always reliable.
2. The rectal mucosa can be entered.

C. Contraindications: Infection at the site of injection.

V. Paracervical Block

Paracervical blockade can be effective for the first stage of labor until the cervix dilates 8 cm or more.

   A. Advantages:
   1. Ease of administration.
   2. Immediate onset of anesthesia.
   B. Disadvantages:
   1. Brief duration.
   2. The need for another technique for delivery.
   3. Fetal bradycardia
   C. Contraindications: Infection at the site of injection.

SUGGESTED READING

Crawford JS. The second thousand epidural blocks, in an obstetric hospital practice. *Br J Anaesth.*, 1972; 44:1277.

Grimes DA, Cates W. Deaths from paracervical anesthesia used for first-trimester abortion. *N Eng J Med.* 1976; 295:1397.

12

General Anesthesia

If regional anesthesia is contraindicated, general anesthesia is to be used for cesarean section.

I. Indications
   A. Uterine relaxation
   B. Maternal hemorrhage
   C. Fetal distress

II. Relative Contraindications
   A. Respiratory disease
   B. Difficult intubation
   C. Sickle cell disease

III. Complications
   A. Aspiration of vomitus
   B. Fetal depression

IV. Advantages
   A. More reliable anesthesia for cesarean section
   B. Control of airway and rapid onset of anesthesia

V. Technique
   A. The patient should be placed in a left lateral tilt on the operating table. Preoxygenation should occur before induction. If an

emergency cesarean section must be done under general anesthesia, the patient should be encouraged to take three deep breaths. Induction of general anesthesia should not occur until the abdomen has been prepped and draped, and when the obstetricians are ready to begin. Cricoid pressure should be applied while laryngoscopy and the intubation is performed. The cuff should be inflated and breath sounds and end tidal CO_2 should be verified before removing cricoid pressure. At that time, 50% O_2 and 50% N_2O may be instituted. Once the intubating dose of succinylcholine has lost its pharmacological effect, as noted by nerve stimulator, a continuous infusion of succinylcholine may be initiated. Before delivery, 0.5% halothane, 0.75% isoflurane, or 1% ethrane may be used until delivery. At that time, a balanced technique may be used. If inhalational agents are to be used throughout surgery, one should not increase the concentrations above the previously mentioned concentrations to prevent uterine relaxation and bleeding.

VI. Induction Techniques

A. Ketamine 1 mg/kg should be used in parturients who are hypovolemic.

B. Induction with 4 mg/kg of thiopental and succinylcholine 1.5 mg/kg should be administered at the beginning of a contraction.

C. The use of curare for defasciculation is controversial. Curare may prolong the onset time of succinylcholine. Furthermore, it has been shown that increases in lower esophageal pressure are greater than increases in intragastric pressure, which theoretically may prevent silent aspiration. If difficulty in intubation is anticipated, one should refer to the chapter on failed intubation.

VII. Oxytocin Infusion

A concentrated infusion of oxytocin may result in intraoperative hypotension. For this reason, one should dilute 20 units of oxytocin in 1 liter of Ringer's lactate solution.

VIII. Extubation

Extubation should occur only after the patient is awake and able to protect her airway.

SUGGESTED READING

Abboud TK, Kim SH, Henriksen EH et al. Comparative maternal and neonatal effects of halothane, enflurane, and isoflurane for cesarean delivery. *Acta Anaesth Scand.* 1985; 29:663.

Finster M, Poppers PJ. Safety of thiopental used for induction of general anesthesia in elective cesarean section. *Anesthesiology.* 1968; 29:190.

Munson ES, Embro WY, Enflurane, isoflurane and halothane and isolated human uterine muscle. *Anesthesiology.* 1977; 46:11.

Warren TM, Daha S, Ostheimer GW. et al. Comparison of the maternal and neonatal effects of halothane, enflurane and isoflurane for cesarean delivery. *Anesth Analg.* 1983; 162:516.

SECTION V

Intrapartum and Postpartum Assessment
and Management of the Fetus
and Newborn

13

Uterine and Fetal Monitoring

I. General Considerations
The most important indices to fetal health are the fetal heart rate (FHR) patterns associated with the patient's uterine contractions. Beat-to-beat recordings are important. Loss of beat-to-beat irregularity may be a sign of fetal compromise.

II. Indications
Fetal monitoring should be used if the patient has a positive cardiovascular history (including hypertension), a previous cesarean section, multiple pregnancies, uterine bleeding, meconium-stained amniotic fluid, or a prolonged first or second stage of labor.

III. Evaluation of Uterine Monitoring

A. Uterine contractions (active labor)
1. The **frequency** is the number of contractions per 10-minute intervals (3 to 4 contractions per 10 minutes is the average in active labor).
2. The **intensity** is the pressure generated

with each uterine contraction; normal is 50 to 100 mm Hg.

3. Tonus is the pressure recorded between contractions. The average pressure is 10 to 20 mm Hg.

4. In early labor, contractions occur every 4 to 5 minutes and last 60 to 70 seconds.

5. As labor progresses, they occur every 2 to 3 minutes and last 80 to 90 seconds.

6. The **peak** of the uterine concentration shuts off fetal venous outflow and maternal arterial inflow.

7. Uterine contractions interfere with intervillous blood flow.

8. Uterine contractions can put pressure on the fetal head, body, or umbilical cord, which can have an effect on the FHR, resulting in early deceleration.

B. Intrauterine pressure baseline
   1. Latent labor: 5 mm Hg
   2. Active phase: 12 mm Hg
   3. Second stage: 20 mm Hg

C. Uterine contraction pattern
   1. Normal: Bell shape with return to baseline
   2. Coupling: Contractions occurring together with a return to baseline
   3. Tetanic contraction: Pressure well above baseline without any or little decrease in the contraction

D. Uterine hyperactivity can develop from excessive oxytocin stimulation or abruptio placenta.

IV. Fetal Monitoring

A. Indirect (external) monitor

1. An **ultrasound transducer** is applied to maternal abdominal wall to monitor fetal heart rate and uterine contractions.

2. In **obese patients,** monitoring may be inaccurate.

3. Ultrasound detection of the FHR may be irregular depending on the signal from the transducer. The ultrasound transducer may pick up artifact, which makes it difficult on occasion to interpret changes in FHR irregularity. It is furthermore difficult to interpret uterine contractions on occasion.

B. Direct (internal) monitor

1. **Uterine activity** is measured by a small fluid-filled catheter introduced transcervically. It is inserted when the cervix is dilated 2 cm and when rupture of the membranes has occurred.

2. It is used by the obstetrician when using uterotonic agents, when the external tracing is poor, when the patient is obese, and when accurate recordings of uterine contractions are necessary for the diagnosis of failure to progress.

C. Evaluation of fetal monitoring

1. **Indirect (external) monitor** is the same as is used for fetal monitoring.

   a. The **Doppler test** is the most commonly used.

   b. **Abdominal fetal ECG** unsuitable in labor because of abdominal muscle activity.

2. Direct (internal) monitor

    a. A spiral electrode is attached to the baby's scalp and allows for direct measurement of the fetal ECG.

    b. Fetal scalp infection is rare.

3. FHR characteristics

    a. The **baseline FHR** is the rate between contractions and 120 to 160 bpm is considered normal.

    b. One must observe the FHR for 15 minutes or longer and establish the variability (normal is 120 to 160 bpm).

    c. Tachycardia (greater than 160 bpm) can be caused by:

        (1) Fever (most common cause)

        (2) Hypoxia (most concerning cause)

        (3) Beta-sympathomimetic agents

        (4) Maternal hyperthyroidism

        (5) Fetal hypovolemia

    d. Bradycardia (less than 120 bpm) can be caused by the following:

        (1) Hypoxia

        (2) Complete heart block

        (3) Beta blockers

        (4) Local anesthetics

        (5) Hypothermia

4. Beat-to-beat variability is the moment-to-moment change in FHR.

    a. It is caused by a balance between the sympathetic stimulation of FHR and parasympathetic suppression of FHR.

    b. Types:

        (1) Short-term (beat-to-beat variability)

(2) Long term (irregular sine waves with a cycle of 3 to 6/minute)

c. **Normal variability** is associated with a normal fetal pH and is associated with fetal well-being.

d. **Decreased variability** is caused by chronic injury or depression of the CNS, fetal hypoxia, acidosis, sleep, narcotics, vagal blockage (atropine), complete heart block, or magnesium sulfate.

e. **Increased variability** may be seen with maternal activity, uterine contractions, and palpation of the uterus.

5. **Periodic changes in FHR**
   a. This occurs in association with the uterine contractions.
   b. Types:
      (1) **Early decelerations (Fig. 13—1)**
         (a) They begin near the onset of the uterine contraction.
         (b) They are caused by head compression (vagal stimulation).
         (c) They mirror the pattern of the uterine contraction.
         (d) They are benign in most instances.
         (e) They are uniform in shape.
      (2) **Late decelerations (Fig. 13—2)**
         (a) They begin as the uterine contraction reaches its peak.
         (b) They are caused by decreased intervillous blood flow (check for hypotension after an epidural or

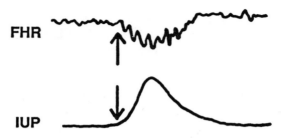

Figure 13–1. EARLY DECELERATION. (1) Specific, uniform FHR pattern whose shape reflects the shape of the associated uterine contraction curve. (2) The onset of the deceleration begins early in the contracting phase of the uterus. (3) Usually does not fall below 100 bpm. (4) Usually of less than 90 seconds' duration. (5) Usually associated with a baseline FHR in the normal range. (6) Probably due to increased pressure on the fetal vertex. (7) Not affected by maternal hyperoxia. (8) Markedly modified by atropine administration. (9) Not associated with changes in fetal acid-base status.

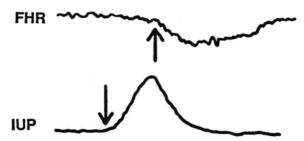

Figure 13–2. LATE DECELERATION. (1) Uniform specific FHR pattern whose shape reflects the shape of the associated uterine contraction curve. (2) The onset of this deceleration is late in the contracting phase of the uterus. (3) Usually decrease in the range of 15–45 bpm, but when severe may be decreased by more than 45 bpm. (4) Usually of less than 90 seconds' duration. (5) Usually associated with a baseline FHR in the high normal or tachycardia range. (6) Probably due to uteroplacental insufficiency. (7) Markedly altered by maternal hyperoxia. (8) Partially modified by atropine administration. (9) Associated with fetal acidosis, when persistent or severe.

aortocaval compression). They may also be seen with hypertension, diabetes mellitus, preeclampsia, or intrauterine growth retardation.

(c) They mirror the pattern of the uterine contraction.

(d) They may be associated with uterine hyperstimulation or abruptio placenta.

(e) They are severe when the FHR drops more than 45 beats below baseline.

(f) They are uniform in shape.

(g) They reflect inadequate fetal reserves. Therefore, the fetus is unable to maintain adequate oxygenation and a normal pH in the face of a decreased intervillous blood flow. It is an ominous pattern.

6. Variable decelerations (Fig. 13–3):

 a. They are nonuniform in shape with a jagged wave form.

 b. They can be caused by cord compression.

 c. They can be seen in the second stage of labor.

 d. They are usually abrupt in onset and cessation.

 e. They are severe when the FHR is below 70 bpm and are longer than 60 seconds.

7. Accelerations with contractions

 a. No prognostic significance is noted

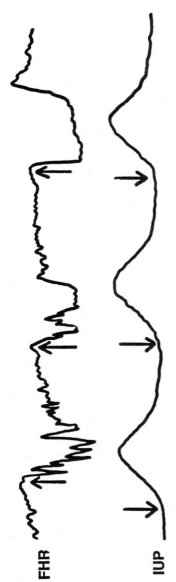

FHR

IUP

Figure 13–3. VARIABLE DECELERATION. (1) It varies markedly in shape from contraction to contraction, and does not reflect the shape of the associated uterine contraction curve. (2) The onset of the deceleration bears a variable time-relationship to the beginning of the associated uterine contraction. (3) It usually falls below 100 bpm and is frequently as low as 50–60 bpm or less. (4) The duration of the deceleration varies from a few seconds to minutes. (5) It is usually associated with a baseline FHR in the normal, or low normal range. (6) It is probably due to umbilical cord occlusion. (7) It is markedly altered by maternal position change or fetal manipulation. (8) It does not appear to be altered by maternal hyperoxia. (9) It is markedly altered by atropine administration. (10) It is not associated with fetal acidosis unless frequent and prolonged.

100

when they occur.
   b. They can be associated with fetal movement.
8. Other patterns
   a. Prolonged decelerations
      (1) Prolonged decelerations are a drop in FHR greater than 30 bpm and lasting 90 to 120 seconds.
      (2) They may be seen with sudden maternal hypotension, cord prolapse, or with tetanic uterine contractions.
   b. Sinusoidal heart rate pattern
      (1) It is a sine wave pattern with a frequency of 4 to 8 cycles/minute.
      (2) The sinusoidal heart rate pattern may be seen with severe fetal anemia (ie, erythroblastosis fetalis).
   c. Sinister heart rate patterns are seen with absent heart rate variability with periodic changes (late or variable decelerations) that are severe in nature.
D. Antepartum fetal monitoring
   1. The **non-stress test** (NST) is an appraisal of fetal well-being based upon the observation that a healthy fetus produces certain FHR patterns but that a fetus in jeopardy does not.
      a. In this test, fetal movements are associated with brief increases in the FHR.
      b. A reactive test is predictive of fetal well-being.
      c. If the test is nonreactive, a repeat test should be done in 24 hours.

2. Stress test—oxytocin challenge test (OCT)

   a. In this test, oxytocin is infused until contractions occur with a duration of 40 to 60 seconds and a frequency of 3 per 10 minutes.

   b. A positive test is defined as late decelerations occurring with 50% of the contractions.

   c. A negative test is defined as no late decelerations occurring.

   d. An equivocal test is defined as late decelerations that occur with less than 50% of the contractions. It should be repeated in 24 hours.

   e. Absent FHR variability that is present with late decelerations is an ominous sign.

   f. When the OCT is positive, 10% of the fetuses may die within 1 week if not delivered.

3. Anesthetic considerations:

   a. If signs of fetal distress are present or if the fetus is hypoxic and acidotic, one may wish to use chloroprocaine if an epidural block is anticipated because of the potential for fetal ion trapping with amide local anesthetics.

   b. With signs of fetal distress, one must avoid any decrease in the maternal blood pressure.

   c. One must minimize aortocaval compression by keeping a wedge under the patient's right side.

d. One should administer oxygen to the mother when fetal distress is noted.

SUGGESTED READING

Hon EH. The electronic evaluation of the fetal heart rate. *Am J Obstet Gynecol.* 1958; 75:1215.

Martin CB. Physiology and clinical use of fetal heart rate variability. *Clin Perinatol.* 1982; 9:339.

Sachs BP, Friedman EA. Antepartum and intrapartum assessment of the fetus: Current status and does it influence outcome? In: Ostheimer GW (ed): *Clinics in Anesthesiology,* Vol 4. London: Saunders Co. p.53, 1986.

Thacker SB, Berkelman SB. Assessing the diagnostic accuracy and efficacy of selected antepartum surveillance techniques. *Obstet Gynecol Surv.* 1986; 41:121.

14

Newborn Resuscitation

I. Initial Evaluation

A. The Apgar score is useful in identifying and treating the depressed neonate. It is measured at 1 and 5 minutes (Apgar, 1953 and 1962).

PARAMETER	Apgar Score		
	0	1	2
Heart rate	0	< 100/min	> 100/min
Respiratory effort	Absent	Slow, irregular	Crying
Reflex irritability	No response	Grimace	Cry
Muscle tone	Limp	Flexion of extremities	Active
Color	Pale/cyanotic	Body pink; Extremities cyanotic	Pink

B. With **scores of 7 or above,** the neonates are normal or have a mild respiratory acidosis. Scores of 4 to 6 indicate a moderately depressed infant who frequently improves with oxygen administered by mask. With a score of 3 or less, intubation and external cardiac massage are indicated (heart rate less than 60).

C. When **scores are 6 or less,** one should obtain additional scores every 5 minutes for 20 minutes.

D. Some helpful **laboratory values:**

1. Fetal capillary pH

- ≥ 7.25 normal
- 7.20–7.24 preacidotic
- < 7.20 acidotic

2. Normal blood gases

	AT BIRTH	AT 30 MIN
P_{O_2}	60	68
P_{CO_2}	40	35
pH	7.25	7.33

II. Suction

1. When thick meconium or bleeding occurs, the neonatal trachea must be suctioned before ventilation.

2. Meconium can be removed from the trachea by inserting an endotracheal tube and aspirating through it as it is withdrawn from the trachea.

III. Drugs Useful in the Resuscitation of the Neonate

A. Atropine (0.03 mg/kg IV or ET tube) for bradycardia

B. Epinephrine (0.1 mL/kg IV or ET tube; 1:10,000 solution) for asystole

C. Calcium chloride (10 to 20 mg/kg IV) for low cardiac output

D. Isoproterenol (4 mg/250 mL; titrate until

heart rate increases; usually 16 μg/kg/ minute) for persistent bradycardia

E. Sodium bicarbonate (1 to 2 mEq/kg)

1. Use if Apgar score is 2 or less at 2 minutes.

2. Very hypertonic and may also induce hypotension.

3. When able to obtain blood gases:

a. If the pH is less than 7, then 1/4 of the base deficit should be corrected with bicarbonate.

b. If the pH is >7.10, the patient should be ventilated and an arterial blood gas (ABG) measured at 5 minutes.

c. If repeat pH shows a decrease or no change, then 1/4 of the base deficit should be corrected.

d. The dose to correct 1/4 of the base deficit is determined by:

$$0.6 \times \text{weight (kg)} \times \text{base deficit.}$$

F. Lidocaine (1 mg/kg) for ventricular arrhythmias

IV. Metabolic Acidosis

A. Occurs because of poor tissue perfusion

B. Can be caused by hypovolemia or heart failure

1. Heart failure can occur when the pH is less than 7.0.

2. Heart failure can be caused by cardiac disease wherein one should begin an isoproterenol drip or insert a transvenous pacemaker.

3. Heart failure may be caused by hypoglycemia, which should be corrected to 45 to 90 mg.

V. Defibrillation and Cardiac Compression

   A. An **energy level** of 2 joules/kg should be used for defibrillation.

   A second attempt may be made at 4 joules/kg (ventricular fibrillation is rare in this age group).

   B. External cardiac compression is best done with both hands encircling the infant's chest with the thumbs used for cardiac compression.

   C. The **rate of compression** should be 100/minute. The depth of compression should be 1/2 to 1 inch.

VI. Equipment

   A. Must be **available in the delivery room** and should include a small diameter laryngoscope handle, 0 and 00 straight blades, endotracheal tubes ranging in size from 2.5 to 3.5 mm, and suction catheters.

   B. Blood gases must be able to be measured immediately.

   C. Heating lamps must be available to maintain a normal body temperature.

VII. Hypovolemia

   A. Neonates may be hypovolemic, which may be caused by placental abruption if their umbilical cord is clamped early or if the cord is tightly wound around the neck and must be cut to expedite delivery.

   B. Hypovolemic neonates are usually pale and have poor capillary refill.

   C. A Doppler measurement of the blood pressure may be helpful in managing the newborn.

D. In the first hour of life, the following blood pressures are considered to be in a normal range, which is dependent on birth weight:

1. 2000 grams: 49 systolic; 35 diastolic

2. 2000 to 3000 grams: 59 systolic; 43 diastolic

3. 3000 grams: 70 systolic; 53 diastolic

E. Hypovolemia should be treated with intravascular volume expansion; one must take care not to overexpand the intravascular volume.

F. One must remember that hypotension can also be caused by hypoglycemia, hypocalcemia, and hypermagnesemia.

SUGGESTED READING

Benitz WE, Sunshine P. Neonatal resuscitation. In: Nelson NM. *Current Therapy in Neonatal-Perinatal Medicine*. Philadelphia, PA: BC Decker Inc. p. 360, 1986.

Gregory GA, Gooding C, Phibbs RH, et al. Meconium aspiration in infants. A prospective study. *J Pediatr*. 1974; 85:848.

SECTION VI

High-Risk Labor and Delivery

15

Anesthetic Considerations for the Patient with Preterm Labor

I. Incidence
Preterm birth occurs in 7 to 10% of all births. Preterm birth accounts for more than 75% of perinatal mortality in the United States.

II. General Considerations
A. Preterm delivery is any delivery occurring before 37 weeks' gestation or when the newborn weight is less than 2500 grams.

B. The etiology of the onset of labor is unknown.

C. Contractile events appear related to increased concentration of free intracellular calcium.

D. Once labor is initiated, progressive labor is associated with increased uteroplacental production of prostaglandins.

E. Preterm labor is common following spontaneous premature rupture of the membranes.

F. Many preterm labors are associated with placental abruptio, uterine anomalies, multiple gestation, urinary infection, and iatrogenic causes.

G. Preterm labor is more prevalent in the low socioeconomic classes.

III. Clinical Findings

A. Tocolysis is most frequent when uterine contractions occur without cervical dilatation.

B. Once cervical dilatation begins to occur, the success of tocolysis is decreased.

IV. Obstetric Management

A. Contraindications to tocolysis include the following:

  1. Uterine infection

  2. Hypertension

  3. Advanced labor

B. Management: Bedrest and rapid infusion of lactated Ringer's solution may be effective in stopping labor.

C. The most widely used pharmacological agents are ethanol, magnesium sulfate, and beta agonists.

D. Ethanol suppresses oxytocin and vasopressin release from the mother and fetus.

E. Side effects include nausea or emesis, inebriation, and metabolic acidosis. For these reasons, ethanol is rarely used.

F. Magnesium sulfate

  1. Magnesium sulfate acts as an antagonist to calcium.

  2. Magnesium sulfate is most effective if the cervix has not dilated more than 2 cm.

  3. A level of 4 to 8 mEq/L is desirable.

  4. Side effects

    a. Hypotension secondary to vasodilation

    b. Interaction with both depolarizing and non-depolarizing muscle relaxants

    c. Respiratory depression

    d. Pulmonary edema
  5. Treatment of magnesium sulfate overdose consists of 10 mL of 10% intravenous calcium gluconate.

G. Beta agonists

  1. Beta agonists may also inactivate intracellular calcium.
  2. Ritodrine (Yutopar) is the only beta agonist that is FDA approved.
  3. Isoxsuprine (Vasodilan) and terbutaline (Brethine) at present lack FDA approval.
  4. Terbutaline and ritodrine are more beta-2 specific than isoxsuprine.
  5. Beta-1 activity is manifest as an increase in the heart rate and the force of contractility.
  6. Beta-2 activity relaxes smooth muscle.
  7. Therapy with beta agonists is with an intravenous infusion. After contractions stop, the patients may be maintained on oral agents.
  8. Side effects of beta agonists include:
    a. Tachycardia
    b. Decreased systemic vascular resistance
    c. Arrhythmias
    d. Hypokalemia
    e. Pulmonary edema
    f. Anxiety
    g. Nausea or emesis
  9. Etiology of pulmonary edema
    a. Pulmonary edema is often associated with prehydration.
    b. Pulmonary edema may be related to increased pulmonary capillary permeability.

10. Treatment of beta agonist pulmonary edema is as follows:
   a. Discontinue the beta agonist.
   b. Administer oxygen.
   c. Check the plasma potassium level.
   d. Administer furosemide.
   e. Check the patient's arterial blood gas.
   f. Occasionally, patients may require intubation and invasive monitoring.
11. Contraindications to beta agonists are:
   a. Heart disease
   b. Hyperthyroidism
   c. Cerebral ischemia
   d. Hypovolemia
   e. Maternal infection
12. Steroid use in preterm labor
   a. Betamethasone or dexamethasone may be administered to attempt to improve fetal lung maturation.
   b. Steroids may increase the incidence of maternal and neonatal infection.
   c. Any patient who is taking steroids should have a sterile dressing placed over the epidural catheter to attempt to minimize infection.
   d. When steroids are used with beta agonists, the incidence of maternal hyperglycemia and pulmonary edema may be increased.

V. Anesthetic Considerations
   A. One must try to avoid induction of general anesthesia for 30 minutes once the beta agonists are discontinued.
   B. Halothane should not be used when a patient

is receiving beta agonists because of the potential for arrhythmias.

C. If a patient receives general anesthesia, hyperventilation should be avoided because it may lower the maternal plasma potassium.

D. One must minimize neonatal depression with pharmacological agents.

E. The premature infant may not have the ability to metabolize or excrete drugs.

F. The premature fetus does not tolerate intrauterine hypoxia.

G. All mothers of preterm infants must have supplemental oxygen.

H. Left uterine displacement must be maintained.

I. Maternal hypotension must be treated immediately if it occurs.

J. Fetal monitoring must be done throughout labor.

K. Maternal hemorrhage can occur because of the increased incidence of abruption and uterine abnormalities associated with preterm labor. Therefore, blood must be readily available.

L. Approximately 28% of preterm deliveries are breech.

M. There is an increased incidence of cesarean sections in the patient with preterm labor because of the following:
   1. Fetal distress
   2. Maternal hemorrhage
   3. Breech presentation

N. Anesthesia for vaginal delivery:
   1. A continuous lumbar epidural block is ideal because, with the continuous tech-

nique, neural blockade can be rapidly extended for an emergency cesarean section. For this reason, a T8 level should be maintained with the continuous lumbar epidural infusion.

   2. Maternal pushing must be minimized to decrease trauma to the fetal head.
   3. A cesarean section may be of benefit in patients who have very low-birth-weight infants (<1500 g). The very low-birth-weight infant may be vulnerable to minimal traumatic events. Consequently, a cesarean section may be of benefit to the fetus.

O. Anesthesia for cesarean section:
   1. A subarachnoid block or lumbar epidural may be done for cesarean section.
   2. The lumbar epidural offers an advantage of postoperative pain relief.
   3. With either block, a minimum level of T4 must be attained.

P. Emergent situations
   1. In emergency situations, a general anesthetic may become necessary.
   2. One must maintain a high FIO_2 until delivery of the baby.
   3. Magnesium sulfate may cause sensitivity to both depolarizing and non-depolarizing muscle relaxants.
   4. For this reason, it is not recommended that one pretreat with curare.
   5. Hyperventilation must be avoided to minimize hypokalemia.
   6. One must be vigilant for tachycardia and

arrhythmias if the patient was receiving beta agonists.

7. Because beta agonists can decrease the maternal systemic vascular resistance, one must be aware that these patients may develop hypotension.

8. Ketamine should be avoided in these patients if possible because of the potential for increased sympathetic tone.

9. If hypotension occurs, the danger of uterine artery vasoconstriction following administration of phenylephrine may be minimal.

10. Ephedrine remains the first drug of choice for the treatment of hypotension.

11. If, however, the patient is receiving a beta agonist and exhibits significant tachycardia, one may wish to administer phenylephrine in 50-μg increments for the correction of hypotension.

12. Following delivery, patients who were receiving tocolytics should be observed for uterine atony.

SUGGESTED READING

Anderson KE, Bengtsson LP, Gustafson I, et al. The relaxing effect of terbutaline on the human uterus during term labor. *Am J Obstet Gynecol.* 1975; 121:602.

Freditzen MC. Tocolytic therapy with beta-adrenergic agonists. *Ration Drug Ther.* 1983; 17:1.

Gibbs CE. Diagnosis and treatment of uterine conditions that may cause prematurity. *Clin Obstet Gynecol.* 1973; 16:159.

Gravett MG. Causes of preterm delivery. *Semin Perinatol.* 1984; 8:246.

Howie PW, Patel NB. Obstetric management of preterm labour. *Clin Obstet Gynaecol.* 1984; 11:373.

Wheeler AS, Patel KF, Spain J. Pulmonary edema during beta-tocolytic therapy. *Anesth Analg.* 1981; 60:695.

16

Anesthetic Considerations for the Patient with a Multiple Gestation

I. Incidence
The incidence of multiple pregnancy is 1/89 deliveries.

II. General Considerations
   A. Multiple pregnancy carries the risk of increased perinatal morbidity and mortality.
   B. Prematurity accounts for the greatest increase in perinatal mortality.

III. Clinical Findings
   A. The uterus is large for the estimated gestation.
   B. A definitive diagnosis is made by ultrasonic scan.

IV. Obstetric Management
   A. If the first twin is breech, a cesarean section may be necessary.
   B. If gestation is less than 32 weeks, a cesarean section may be necessary.
   C. With vertex presentation of the first twin, a trial of labor may be attempted and the indica-

tions for cesarean section are the same as for a singleton pregnancy.

D. Uterine atony can occur postoperatively.

V. Anesthetic Considerations

A. One must be ready to administer a general anesthetic with endotracheal anesthesia using an inhalational agent to relax the uterus if necessary. This applies to both vaginal delivery and cesarean section.

B. Epidural analgesia should be done with 0.25% bupivacaine to enable the mother to preserve motor function. Rapid epidural anesthesia can be established with 3% 2-chloroprocaine carbonated to a pH of 7.7 (3 mL of 8.4% $NaHCO_3$/27 mL 3% 2CP).

C. One must be observant for aortocaval compression.

D. Good perineal anesthesia is necessary if a premature breech presentation is to be delivered.

SUGGESTED READING

Ackerman W, Juneja MM, Denson DD, et al. The effect of pH and pCO_2 on the onset of epidural 2CP. *Anesth Analg.* 1989; 61:S5.

Chervenak FA, Johnson RE, Yocha S, et al. Intrapartum management of twin gestation. *Obstet Gynecol.* 1985; 65:119.

Hawrylyshyn PA, Barkin M, Bernstein A et al. Twin pregnancies: A continuing perinatal challenge. *Obstet Gynecol.* 1982; 59:463.

17

Anesthetic Considerations for the Patient with Abruptio Placenta

I. Incidence
Abruptio placenta accounts for 30% of antepartum bleeding and the incidence is 1/200 pregnancies.

II. General Considerations
  A. Two types are recognized:
  1. **Internal,** which consists of painful hemorrhage without external bleeding.
  2. **External,** painless hemorrhage with bleeding through the cervix.

  B. It usually occurs after the 23rd week.

  C. Abruptio placenta occurs in 50% of patients before the onset of labor and in 10 to 15% of patients during the second stage of labor.

  D. Approximately 80% of patients are multiparous.

  E. Approximately 66% of patients have pre-eclampsia.

III. Clinical Findings
  A. Classification

1. **Grade 0** (30%): No signs or symptoms are noted; it is recognized after delivery.
2. **Grade 1** (45%): External bleeding occurs but uterine tetany and uterine pain are not present; there is no fetal distress.
3. **Grade 2** (15%): Uterine tetany and pain occur; fetal distress is present.
4. **Grade 3** (10%): Uterine tetany is marked; maternal shock, coagulation defects, and fetal death occur.

B. Signs and symptoms:
   1. Patients with external bleeding usually have no pain.
   2. Patients with concealed hemorrhage can have considerable pain.
   3. The patients may have severe back pain.
   4. The uterus fails to relax.
   5. Fetal distress will be apparent on fetal monitoring.
   6. Anemia and coagulation problems may be noted.
   7. Ultrasound may be helpful in making a diagnosis.

IV. Obstetric Management

   A. Clotting must be restored to normal before delivery.
   B. A cesarean section may be required if the patient is in severe fetal distress.
   C. After delivery, coagulation factors usually return to normal in 24 hours while platelets return to normal in 2 to 4 days.

V. Anesthetic Considerations

   A. Two large bore intravenous lines must be started.

B. Fluid and blood must be replaced as indicated.

C. A vaginal delivery may be done if the mother and infant are stable or if intrauterine fetal death occurred.

D. A cesarean section is usually performed for maternal or fetal distress.

E. Regional anesthesia can be done in Grade 0 and Grade 1 patients (mild).

F. Ketamine should be used as an induction agent for general anesthesia in the hypovolemic patient. Ketamine will not cause further uterine tetany at <1 mg/kg.

SUGGESTED READING

Abdella EJ, Baha, M.S, Hays JM, et al. Relationship of hypertensive disease to abruptio placenta. *Obstet Gynecol.* 1984; 63:365.

Notelovitz M, Bottoms SF, Dase DF, et al. Painless abruptio placentae. *Obstet Gynecol.* 1978; 53:270.

Sher G. Pathogenesis and management of uterine inertia complicating abruptio placentae with consumption coagulopathy. *Am J Obstet Gynecol.* 1977; 129:164.

18

Anesthetic Considerations for the Patient with Placenta Previa

I. Incidence

    A. Placenta previa is more common among older women.

    B. The incidence of placenta previa is 1/200 pregnancies.

II. General Considerations

    A. In placenta previa, the placenta obstructs the descent of the presenting part, as the placenta develops within the lower uterine segment.

    B. The etiology is unknown. Tumors, scars from previous surgery, and conditions associated with impaired vascularization of the decidua may be causes.

    C. Types of placenta previa:

        1. Partial: Only part of the internal os is covered (30%).

        2. Complete: The internal os is covered (45%).

        3. Marginal: The edge of the placenta is at the os but does not cover the os (25%).

III. Clinical Findings:

A. Painless uterine bleeding is the principal symptom.

B. Marked bleeding usually begins after the 28th week of gestation.

C. An occasional contraction may be noted, which may cause bleeding.

D. Bleeding is bright red in color.

E. Bleeding is due to mechanical separation of the placenta from the uterus.

IV. Obstetric Management

A. Breech presentations are common with placenta previa.

B. Ultrasonography may help in the diagnosis of placenta previa. The degree of coverage of the os can only be approximated.

C. Double set-up: The patient is prepped for an emergency cesarean section. A vaginal examination will be performed by the obstetrician and, if hemorrhage occurs, a rapid sequence-controlled induction of anesthesia should follow.

D. Placenta previa is more common in previous cesarean sections.

E. The FHR should be monitored throughout labor because the fetus is at risk.

F. Three choices of therapy exist:

    1. Expectant treatment consists of bedrest with observation with an ultimate goal of fetal maturity before either vaginal delivery or cesarean section.

    2. Vaginal delivery can be done. If vaginal delivery is contemplated, an **amniotomy** should be done. An amniotomy may allow tamponade of the presenting part against the placental edge, which theoretically can decrease bleeding as labor progresses.

3. If a **cesarean section** is contemplated, the obstetrician should avoid laceration of the placenta.

V. Anesthetic Considerations

A. Each patient should have two large bore intravenous lines upon admission to the labor hall.

B. If the patient is not pre-eclamptic, one should use ketamine (1 mg/kg or less) for induction of general anesthesia.

C. If the patient is not pre-eclamptic, one might consider etomidate instead of thiopental, 0.3 mg/kg, for induction.

D. Uterine contractions can be a major source of hemorrhage. For this reason, some obstetricians may use tocolytic agents to stop labor.

E. If a cesarean section is decided upon, blood and fluid replacement should be done before incision if time permits.

F. Maternal mortality is approximately 0.5%.

G. The perinatal mortality is approximately 15%. Preterm delivery is a major cause of fetal death. The fetus can also die as a result of intrauterine asphyxia.

H. Blood must be available for immediate transfusion.

SUGGESTED READING

McShane PM, Heyl PS, Epstein MF. Maternal and perinatal morbidity resulting from placenta previa. *Obstet Gynecol*. 1985; 65:176.

Silver RD, Depp R, Sabbagha RE, et al. Placenta previa: Aggressive expectant management. *Am J Obstet Gynecol*. 1984; 150:15.

19

Anesthetic Considerations for the Patient with Uterine Rupture

I. Incidence
   A. Spontaneous rupture of an intact uterus can occur during labor.
   B. Uterine rupture can also occur in a previous uterine scar.
   C. It is more common in multiparas.
   D. In approximately 1 to 2% of classic and 0.5 to 1% of low segment incisions, uterine rupture can occur in subsequent pregnancies.
   E. The overall incidence of uterine rupture is 1/500 deliveries in the United States.

II. General Considerations
   A. The classic operation scar usually ruptures suddenly.
   B. The low segment scar usually ruptures incompletely and slowly. The rupture is frequently noticed at repeat cesarean section.

III. Clinical Findings
   A. Rupture of the uterus may be hard to distinguish from abruption.
   B. Pain may vary from mild to severe.

    C. The patients may have mild-to-severe bleeding.

    D. Labor may stop.

    E. There may be loss of fetal movement and heart tones.

    F. Tetanic contractions can occur.

IV. Obstetric Management

    A. The patient must have an immediate abdominal laparotomy with general anesthesia.

    B. Ketamine should be used as the induction agent.

    C. Uterine repair can be attempted or the patient may require a hysterectomy.

    D. Oxytocin may be used in the patient with a previous low segment uterine scar during labor.

    E. Continual fetal heart rate and uterine monitoring must be continuously done throughout labor.

V. Anesthetic Considerations

    A. Abdominal pain is not always a reliable symptom of uterine rupture. For this reason, there is no contraindication to placing an epidural in a patient who had a previous cesarean section.

    B. An epidural block does not increase the risk of uterine rupture when the patient is placed in the lateral position instead of sitting.

    C. The anesthesiologist and obstetrician must be present during labor in the event that a uterine rupture occurs.

    D. One may consider the use of a continuous epidural infusion during labor to a T10 level, which is helpful if an emergency cesarean section must be performed. If severe bleeding occurs, a general anesthetic should be administered with ketamine, 1 mg/kg, as the induction agent.

E. The patient should be cross-matched for blood.

SUGGESTED READING

Carlsson C, Nybell-Lindahl G, Ingemarison I. Extradural block in patients who have previously undergone cesarean section. *Br J Anaesth*. 1980; 52:287.

Lavin JP. Vaginal delivery after cesarean birth: Frequently asked questions. *Clin Perenatol*. 1983; 10:439.

Plauche WC, Von Almen W, Miller R. Catastrophic uterine rupture. *Obstet Gynecol*. 1984; 64:792.

20

Anesthetic Considerations for the Patient with a Retained Placenta

I. Incidence
Retained placenta occurs in 1% of all vaginal deliveries.

II. General Considerations
   A. It should be suspected if bleeding persists without uterine atony.
   B. The placenta should be inspected for wholeness.
   C. Ultrasonography is useful in making the diagnosis.
   D. By definition, retained placenta is failure to deliver the placenta within 30 minutes after delivery.

III. Clinical Findings
   A. Bleeding in the absence of lacerations or atony.
   B. Late postpartum bleeding may be noted.
   C. Ultrasonography may be helpful in making a diagnosis.

IV. Obstetric Management
   A. The placenta or placental fragments may be removed manually.

B. Occasionally, a D&C may be necessary to remove placental fragments.

V. Anesthetic Considerations

A. If an epidural anesthetic has dissipated, it should not be redosed if the patient's cardiovascular status is unstable.

B. The patient's cardiovascular status must be monitored and the appropriate volumes of blood or fluids must be administered.

C. General endotracheal anesthesia should be instituted with intravenous ketamine if the patient is hypovolemic. The dose of ketamine should not exceed 1 mg/kg because higher doses may increase uterine tone, making extraction of the placenta or placental parts difficult. Once the patient is hemodynamically stable, an inhalational agent can be used.

SUGGESTED READING

Galloon S. Ketamine for dilatation and curettage. *Can Anaesth Soc J*. 1971; 18:600.

Oats JN, Vasey DP, Waldron BA, et al. Effects of ketamine on the pregnant uterus. *Br J Anaesth*. 1979; 51:1163.

21

Anesthetic Considerations for the Patient with Uterine Atony

I. Incidence
   A. The incidence will vary depending on the etiology.

   B. Uterine atony may be associated with multiple pregnancy, a large fetus, prolonged labor, failure of the placenta to separate, inhalational anesthesia, retained placental fragments, beta agonists, overdistention of the uterus (ie, twins, hydramnios), inhalational anesthetics, and tocolytics.

II. General Considerations
   A. The failure of the uterus to contract is the basic pathophysiology.

   B. Severe hypotension resulting in hypoxia of uterine musculature can cause uterine atony.

III. Clinical Findings
   A. Persistent uterine bleeding, which may lead to severe hypotension, may occur.

IV. Obstetric Management
   A. Treatment consists of manual massage of the uterus and oxytocin (20 to 40 units/1000 Lactated Ringer's Solution [LR]).

B. Methergine alkaloids (0.2 mg) may be given intramuscularly.

C. Prostaglandin F_2 alpha (0.25) mg has been shown to be beneficial given intramuscularly or 1 mg by intramyometrial injection.

D. Because oxytocin is a vasodilator, hypotension can occur when the infusion is initiated with a concentrated solution. Therefore, the blood pressure must be monitored closely.

E. Exploratory laparotomy may be required with ligation of the uterine arteries. Hypogastric artery ligation may be performed.

F. A hysterectomy may be indicated if bleeding persists in spite of what has been previously mentioned.

G. Four to 6 units of cross-matched blood should be available if a hysterectomy is necessary.

V. Anesthetic Considerations

A. Anesthetic considerations include monitoring of the cardiovascular status and blood replacement.

B. If a general anesthetic must be given, inhalational agents should not be used initially until the patient's plasma volume is corrected.

C. Assess blood loss.

D. Establish adequate intraveous access.

E. Do not redose epidural catheter if the patient is hemodynamically unstable.

F. Induce general anesthesia with 1 mg/kg of ketamine.

G. Maintain anesthesia with fentanyl.

SUGGESTED READING

Hayashi RH, Bruce SL, Paul RN, Van Dorsten JP. Control of postpartum uterine atony by intramyometrial prostaglandin. *Obstet Gynecol* 1982; 59:475.

Hayashi RH, et al. Management of severe postpartum hemorrhage due to uterine atony using an analogue of prostaglandin F_2 alpha. *Obstet Gynecol.* 1981; 58:426.

Pritchard JA. Obstetric hemorrhage. In: Pritchard JA and McDonald PC, eds. *Williams' Obstetrics* Appleton-Century-Crofts, New York, p 398, 1976.

22

Anesthetic Considerations for the Patient with Inversion of the Uterus

Uterine inversion usually occurs just after delivery but can also occur up to several weeks postpartum.

I. Incidence
   The incidence is 1/15,000 deliveries.

II. General Considerations
   A. Etiologies can include traction on the umbilical cord, a vigorous Crede's maneuver, and separation and extraction of a placenta that adheres to the uterus.
   B. Uterine inversion may be partial or complete.

III. Clinical Findings
   A. Bleeding can occur, which can progress to shock.
   B. The patient may complain of abdominal pain.
   C. The obstetrician may not be able to palpate the fundus of the uterus.
   D. Protrusion of the inverted uterus out of the vagina.

IV. Obstetric Management
   A. The uterus is replaced by manual manipulation, which is usually 75% successful.
   B. Deep general anesthesia is usually required for correction of inversion of the uterus.

   C. If manual replacement is not possible, transvaginal or transabdominal replacement may be necessary.
   D. Once the uterus is placed in its normal position, oxytocin or methergine should be given. If the uterus cannot be replaced, a cesarean section must be done.
V. Anesthetic Considerations
   A. General endotracheal anesthesia must be administered following a rapid sequence induction.
   B. The choice of induction agent depends on the patient's hemodynamic status. Ketamine, 1 mg/kg, should be used as the induction agent unless contraindicated.
   C. When reduction is completed, the patient should be hyperventilated to decrease the alveolar concentration of inhalational agent and to decrease uterine bleeding. Bleeding may be profuse. Two large bore intravenous lines should be placed.
   D. Adequate intravenous access must be present.
   E. The patient's blood must be immediately crossmatched.
   F. Atropine, 0.8 mg, administered intravenously may be necessary as vagal stimulation may occur with uterine manipulation.

SUGGESTED READING

Harris BA. Acute puerperal inversion of the uterus. *Clin Obstet Gynecol.* 1984; 27:134.

Wats JE, Watson P, Besch N, et al. Management of acute and subacute puerperal inversion of the uterus. *Obstet Gynecol.* 1980; 55:12.

23

Anesthetic Considerations for the Patient with Abnormal Presentation

Ten percent of deliveries can present with abnormal presentation. Breech, brow, or face presentations may occur.

I. Breech Presentation
 A. Occurs in 3 to 4% of deliveries (4/1000 deliveries).
 B. It is more common with twins, prematurity, and placenta previa.
 C. The fetal buttocks is the presenting part as opposed to the head.
 D. There are three types (Fig. 23–1):
  1. Frank: the extremities are flexed at the hips and extended at the knees.
  2. Complete: One or both knees are flexed as are the hips.
  3. Incomplete: One or both hips extended with a foot or knee in the birth canal.
 E. Obstetric management
  1. The use of cesarean section for breech delivery is increased. Complete and footling breeches should be delivered by cesarean section.
  2. A frank breech may be delivered vaginally.

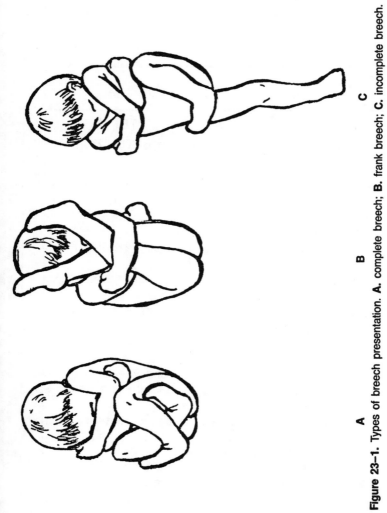

A   B   C

Figure 23–1. Types of breech presentation. **A.** complete breech; **B.** frank breech; **C.** incomplete breech.

146

3. Cesarean section may be performed on all premature breeches because of the increased morbidity associated with vaginal delivery. Furthermore, the cervix can entrap the fetal head during vaginal delivery.

F. Anesthetic considerations

1. The bearing down efforts of the mother must be preserved. If an epidural is used, a low concentration of anesthetic (ie, 0.25% bupivacaine) should be used.

2. If the fetal head is entrapped during vaginal delivery, endotracheal general anesthesia should be performed immediately with 3% halothane with oxygen.

II. Brow Presentation

A. Occurs in 1/1000 deliveries.

B. The diagnosis is made on vaginal examination.

C. The etiology is due to inadequate flexion of the head.

D. Obstetric management

1. Two thirds of these patients convert to a face or occiput presentation.

2. On occasion, a cesarean section may be necessary for delivery.

E. Anesthetic management: An epidural with 0.25% bupivacaine should be sufficient to preserve maternal bearing down efforts.

III. Face Presentation

A. Occurs in 1/500 deliveries.

B. The diagnosis is made on vaginal examination.

C. The etiology is also related to inadequate head flexion during labor.

D. A mentum posterior position usually cannot be delivered vaginally and, in most instances, a cesarean section is indicated.

  E. Anesthetic considerations: An epidural anesthetic that preserves the mother's ability to effectively push should be sufficient.

IV. Occiput Posterior

  A. The incidence of cervical and perineal lacerations is increased during delivery.

  B. A forceps delivery may be necessary.

  C. One should avoid regional anesthetic techniques, which can result in relaxation of the perineal muscles until spontaneous internal rotation of the fetal head occurs.

V. Transverse Lie

  A. Occurs in 1/1200 deliveries.

  B. There is greater frequency associated with multiple gestations and with birth weights less than 1500 g.

  C. A diagnosis is made when a shoulder or arm is palpated upon vaginal examination.

  D. A cesarean section is usually necessary.

  E. Anesthetic considerations:

    1. Either an epidural or subarachnoid block may be done for cesarean section.

    2. Epidural analgesia may be used for labor to provide analgesia before cesarean section.

SUGGESTED READING

Brenner WE, Bruce RD, Hendricks CH. The characteristics and perils of breach presentation. *Am J Obstet Gynecol* 1974; 118:700.

Freidman EA. *Labor: Clinical Evaluation and Management.* 2nd ed, New York, Appleton-Century-Crofts; 1978.

Phelan JP, Stine LE, Edwards NB, et al. The role of external version in the intrapartum management of the transverse lie presentation. *Am J Obstet Gynecol.* 1985; 151:724.

SECTION VII

Coexisting Disease

24

Anesthetic Considerations for the Patient with Neurological Disease

I. Neurological disease is not commonly encountered by the anesthetist during pregnancy. Neurological disease, however, can affect the anesthetic management of the parturient.

    A. Paralysis. With spinal cord lesions above T_7, one must observe for autonomic hyperreflexia. One may observe bradycardia, hypertension, and severe headaches. Contraction of a hollow viscus (ie, uterus) can result in sympathetic nervous system stimulation. Lesions above T_{10} result in painless labor.

        1. Anesthetic considerations. Succinylcholine should be avoided if intubation is necessary. One should use a non-depolarizing muscle relaxer for intubation. Subarachnoid or epidural anesthesia may be used for cesarean section and vaginal delivery and may prevent autonomic hyperreflexia. Treatment of autonomic hyperreflexia includes phentolamine, 2 to 5 mg intravenously (onset of 1 to 2 minutes with a duration of about 10 minutes) or sodium nitroprusside by intravenous infusion beginning at 0.1 mg/kg/minute (immediate onset).

B. Subarachnoid hemorrhage. The incidence of a cerebral hemorrhage during pregnancy is 1/10,000 pregnancies. Subarachnoid hemorrhage accounts for 5 to 24% of maternal deaths. Cerebral aneurysms and arteriovenous (AV) malformations occur with equal frequency. Arteriovenous malformations, if they bleed, usually hemorrhage between 15 and 20 weeks' gestation. Cerebral aneurysms, on the other hand, usually bleed between 30 and 40 weeks' gestation. Arteriovenous malformations have a greater propensity for recurrent bleeding than cerebral aneurysms. Symptoms of subarachnoid hemorrhage can include a severe headache, nausea, and vomiting.

  1. Anesthetic considerations. Cesarean section offers no advantage over vaginal delivery with the exception of an untreated AV malformation, which should have delivery of the fetus performed at 38 weeks' gestation. Delivery by cesarean section under general anesthesia immediately followed by clipping of a ruptured cerebral aneurysm has been reported. For controlled hypotension during neurosurgery in the parturient, trimethaphan has not been shown to harm the fetus. When deliberate hypotension is used for neurosurgery in the pregnant patient, fetal monitoring must be used perioperatively. Coughing and straining on the endotracheal tube during induction and emergence general anesthesia must be avoided.

C. Multiple sclerosis. Multiple sclerosis is characterized by remission and exacerbation and is a demyelinating disease.

1. **Delivery.** The method of delivery of the fetus is determined by obstetric conditions.
2. **Anesthetic considerations.** Regional anesthesia including lumbar puncture does not affect multiple sclerosis. General anesthesia may be used for cesarean section using thiopental, succinylcholine, and inhalational anesthesia.

D. **Myasthenia gravis.** Myasthenia gravis is distinguished by fatigue, muscle wasting, and weakness of the distal and ocular muscles. It is an autoimmune disorder whose incidence is 2:1 in females when compared to males. The disease is an autoimmune disorder with reduced function of acetylcholine receptors.

1. **Anesthetic considerations.** The disease does not affect the course of labor. Anticholinesterase therapy should continue during labor. Magnesium sulfate should be avoided if possible. Epidural or parenteral opioids should be avoided in these patients during labor because anticholinesterases can potentiate opioids. For vaginal delivery, subarachnoid or epidural analgesia can be used. Anticholinesterases may affect the hydrolysis of esters. This must be taken into consideration if one anticipates using ester local anesthesia. For cesarean section, epidural or subarachnoid anesthesia may be used. One, however, must keep the level from becoming too high because impairment of respiratory muscles can occur.

If general anesthesia must be done, curare should not be used before succinylcholine because these patients may be sensitive to curare. Anticholinesterases can result in respiratory tract secretions. Succinylcholine can have an unpredictable effect in these patients. Therefore, a nerve stimulator should be placed before and be used during induction of general anesthesia. The dose of succinylcholine can range from 30 to 60 mg intravenously. Parturients with myasthenia gravis may need ventilatory support postoperatively.

SUGGESTED READING

Abouleish E. Hypertension in a paraplegic parturient. *Anesthesiology*. 1980; 53:348.

Barrett JM, van Hooydenk JE, Boehm FH, et al. Pregnancy-related rupture of arterial aneurysms. *Obstet Gynecol Surv*. 1982; 37:557.

Conklin KA, Herr G, Fung D, et al. Anaesthesia for caesarean section and cerebral aneurysm clipping. *Can Anaesth Soc J*. 1984; 31:451.

Donchin Y, Amirav B, Yarkoni S, et al. Sodium nitroprusside for aneurysm surgery in pregnancy. *Br J Anaesth*. 1978; 50:849.

Newman B, Lam AM. Induced hypotension for clipping of a cerebral aneurysm during pregnancy: A case report and brief review. *Anesth Analg*. 1986; 65:675.

Paterson RA, Tousignant M, Skene DS, et al. Caesarean section for twins in a patient with myotonic dystrophy. *Can Anaesth Soc J*. 1985; 32:418.

Rolbin SH, Levinson G, Schnider SM, et al. Anesthetic considerations for myasthenia gravis and pregnancy. *Anesth Analg*. 1978; 57:44.

Robinson JL, Hall CS, Sedzimir CB, et al. Arteriovenous malformations. Aneurysms and pregnancy. *J Neurosurg*. 1974; 41:63.

Willoughby JS. Sodium nitroprusside, pregnancy and multiple intracranial aneurysms. *Anaesth Intensive Care*. 1984; 12:358.

25

Anesthetic Considerations for the Patient with Pregnancy-Induced Hypertension, Pre-Eclampsia, and Eclampsia

I. The hypertensive diseases of pregnancy have a common denominator, which is an increase in the mean arterial pressure.
- **A. Incidence of hypertension**
    - **1.** 250,000 women become hypertensive during pregnancy.
    - **2.** Hypertension occurs in 7% of pregnancies.
- **B. Effects on neonate:** Pregnancy-induced hypertension can result in prematurity and perinatal death.

II. General Considerations
- **A.** Four categories of hypertension are associated with pregnancy as classified by the American College of Obstetricians and Gynecologists:
    - **1.** Gestational hypertension: Increase in mean arterial pressure after 20 weeks' gestation without proteinuria.
    - **2.** Pre-eclampsia: Hypertension and proteinuria with or without edema.
    - **3.** Chronic hypertension.

4. Chronic hypertension with superimposed pre-eclampsia.

III. Clinical Findings

A. Pre-eclampsia

1. Consists of a triad of hypertension, proteinuria, and edema after 20 weeks' gestation.

2. Pre-eclampsia usually occurs after the 24th week.

3. The incidence is 5 to 7% during pregnancy.

4. It is more frequent at the extreme of childbearing age and in women of lower socioecomonic status.

5. Pre-eclampsia may occur more frequently in patients with underlying chronic hypertension, diabetes mellitus, multiple gestations, and hydatidiform moles.

6. The clotting factors may be decreased in 10 to 20% of pre-eclamptic patients.

7. One should obtain a bleeding time in addition to a coagulation profile (eg, PT, PTT) if there is a marked drop in platelets.

B. Eclampsia

1. Eclampsia occurs if there is the development of seizures or coma in the pre-eclamptic patient.

2. All organs may be affected as follows:

    a. Brain edema and scattered focal hemorrhages can occur.

    b. The liver may develop hemorrhage, thrombosis, and necrosis.

    c. The kidneys may develop hyaline degeneration.

    d. The placenta may be smaller than normal.

    e. Disseminated intravascular coagulation (DIC) may occur.

C. HELLP syndrome is characterized by hemolysis, elevated liver enzymes, and low platelets associated with pre-eclampsia.

D. Severe pre-eclampsia

    1. The following criteria of pre-eclampsia classify pre-eclampsia or severe pre-eclampsia:

        a. A systolic blood pressure of 160 torr, a diastolic pressure of 110 torr.

        b. Proteinuria greater than 5 g/24 hours.

        c. Oliguria as defined as less than 500 mL/ 24 hours.

        d. The above criteria may be seen with headaches, epigastric pain, or pulmonary edema.

E. Etiology is unknown but may include interference with normal activity or involve uteroplacental insufficiency. There is an increased response to angiotensin.

F. Mortality

    1. Maternal mortality may be from cerebral hemorrhages, hepatic rupture, myocardial infarction with subsequent cardiac arrest, or complications from pulmonary edema.

    2. Perinatal mortality may be due to placental infarction or placental growth retardation.

G. Laboratory studies

    1. CBC: Hematocrit may be elevated. If it increases, the intravascular volume may be decreasing.

    2. Liver enzymes should be examined if pre-eclampsia is suspected. Rising values indicate a worsening of the disease.

3. Platelet counts should be monitored daily if less than 100,000/μL.

IV. Obstetric Management

A. Management of hypertension is important in the management of pregnancy-induced hypertension. Methyldopa and hydralazine are effective and have minimal effects on the fetus.

  a. Methyldopa depletes norepinephrine at postganglionic nerve endings. It decreases peripheral arteriolar resistance. The dose is 250 to 500 mg PO q8h. Side effects include hemolytic anemia or elevated liver enzymes.

  b. Hydralazine may be given alone or in combination with methyldopa. Hydralazine directly decreases peripheral arteriolar resistance. The dose is 20 to 40 mg PO q6h.

B. Management of the pre-eclamptic patient

  1. Delivery of the fetus and placenta is the primary therapy of pre-eclampsia.

  2. Pharmacological therapy:

  a. Magnesium sulfate

    (1) First used in 1925 to treat pre-eclampsia.

    (2) It decreases neuromuscular transmission and catecholamine release. It also decreases systemic vascular resistance (SVR).

    (3) Therapeutic plasma levels are 4 to 6 mEq/L. At 7 to 10 mEq/L, there is loss of the patellar reflex. At 12 mEq/L, there may be prolonged AV conduction. Respiratory failure can occur at 14 to 18 mEq/L. Cardiac arrest can occur at 24 mEq/L.

(4) Side effects include potentiation of a neuromuscular block as well as slowing labor by relaxing the uterus. Calcium gluconate is used to reverse the side effects of magnesium sulfate.

b. Sodium nitroprusside

(1) Its use is controversial because of the potential for fetal cyanide toxicity and maternal tachyphylaxis. These effects are rare when used short term.

(2) It is an arterial and venous vasodilator that is rapid acting and has a short duration.

(3) One should limit the dose to 2 μg/kg/minute with infusion limited to 6 hours.

c. Nitroglycerin

(1) It is a venodilator and is used for preload reduction.

(2) Neonatal hypotension has not been observed.

(3) It is used in a dose of 10 μg/kg/minute.

d. Hydralazine

(1) It is the most commonly used vasodilator during labor and can increase uterine blood flow.

(2) It is a direct arterial vasodilator and can be used to decrease the afterload.

(3) Its onset is 15 to 20 minutes.

(4) The dose is 5 to 10 mg every 20 minutes until 20 mg have been given.

(5) It can pass to the fetus and cause fetal hypotension.

(6) It can cause maternal tachycardia.

e. Calcium channel blockers are currently investigational.

f. Labetalol

(1) It has alpha- and beta-blocking properties.

(2) It decreases the blood pressure without decreasing uteroplacental blood flow.

(3) Its effects on the fetus remain to be studied.

g. Methyldopa, diazoxide, and trimethaphan are not commonly used.

3. One should keep the diastolic blood pressure at 90 torr since inadequate uterine perfusion can occur if the blood pressure is lowered too rapidly.

V. Anesthetic Considerations in the Patient with Pre-Eclampsia

A. Epidural

1. A concern to its use is the effect of **hypotension.**

2. Furthermore, fluid bolusing could cause pulmonary edema in certain patients.

3. Slow dosing of local anesthetics can minimize the incidence of hypotension.

4. One must ascertain that the patient does not have a bleeding disorder before initiation of epidural analgesia.

5. If there are signs of fetal distress, the use of 2-chloroprocaine may be prudent because of minimal fetal effects due to its rapid metabolism in the maternal plasma.

B. Subarachnoid block: Because of the rapid onset of a subarachnoid block, it may be prudent to avoid a spinal block because of the potential for hypotension.

C. General anesthesia

   1. It may be necessary in fetal distress.

   2. Ketamine should be avoided.

   3. These patients may have laryngeal edema, consequently one should prepare to use a smaller endotracheal tube.

   4. Both the non-depolarizing and depolarizing muscle relaxants can be potentiated by $MgSO_4$.

   5. One should not administer *d*-tubocurare.

   6. The patient who had a general anesthetic should be carefully observed for 48 hours.

D. Volume replacement: It is controversial whether colloid or crystalloid should be administered.

E. Monitoring

   1. The central venous pressure may not correlate with the pulmonary capillary wedge pressure (PCWP). Therefore, a pulmonary artery catheter may be useful in patients who require vigorous fluids.

   2. Any patient who remains oliguric after a fluid challenge should receive a pulmonary artery catheter.

   3. If patients show signs of pulmonary edema, an arterial line should be placed. Furthermore, if the patient has severe pre-eclampsia, an arterial should be placed.

F. Three subsets of pre-eclampsia

   1. Subset I

      a. One sees a decreased or normal cardiac output with a decreased PCWP and an increased systemic vascular resistance (SVR).

   b. These patients respond to fluids and vasodilators.

2. Subset II:

   a. One may see an increased cardiac output and a normal or decreased SVR.

   b. These patients may be treated with beta blockers and cautious fluid administration.

3. Subset III:

   a. This subset is characterized by a decreased cardiac output, a normal or increased PCWP, and an increased SVR.

   b. These patients respond to fluid restriction and arterial vasodilation.

G. Colloid osmotic pressures (COP): Patients with pregnancy-induced hypertension may have a lower COP (17 mm Hg) than normal (22 to 24 mm Hg).

H. Eclamptic seizures

   1. One should treat the patient with **oxygen** and **anticonvulsant medications.**

   2. Diazepam or **thiopental** can be used.

   3. Thiopental (50 to 150 mg) may be preferred to diazepam because diazepam crosses the placenta and has a longer elimination half-life in the fetus.

   4. Succinylcholine must be available if one has difficulty in maintaining an airway and must intubate the patient.

I. Laboratory tests: The following laboratory tests can be useful: CBC, coagulation profile (platelet count, fibrinogen level, PT and PTT), liver function tests, a renal profile, serum electrolytes, serum glucose, and ABG if indicated.

HEMODYNAMIC VALUES IN HEALTHY PREGNANT AND NONPREGNANT SUBJECTS

PARAMETER	NONPREGNANT	Trimester		
		1ST	2ND	3RD
Heart rate (beat/min)	60–100	81	82	84
Mean arterial pressure (mm Hg)	90–110	82	84	86
Cardiac output (L/min)	4.3–6.0	6.2	6.3	6.4
Stroke volume (mL/beat)	57–71	76	75	76
Systemic vascular resistance (dynes x s x cm^{-5})	900–1400	1087	1093	1119

SUGGESTED READING

Clark SH, Greenspoon JJ, Aldahl D, et al. Severe preeclampsia with persistent oliguria. Management of hemodynamic subsets. *Am J Obstet Gynecol*. 1987; 154:491.

Cotton DB, Benedetti TJ. Use of the Swan-Ganz catheter in obstetrics and gynecology. *Obstet Gynecol*. 1980; 56:641.

Morrison D. Continuing medical education article: Anesthesia and pre-eclampsia. *Can J Anaesth*. 1987; 34:415.

Shnider S, Levinson G. *Anesthesia for Obstetrics*. 2nd ed. Baltimore: Williams & Wilkins; 1987; 225–240.

26

Anesthetic Considerations for the Patient with Diabetes Mellitus

I. **Incidence:** The incidence in pregnancy is 1 in 300 pregnancies (the incidence is increased with parity).

II. **General Considerations**
   A. Diabetes is a metabolic disorder caused by a relative or absolute lack of insulin.
   B. Reduced insulin production or decreased sensitivity to insulin affects carbohydrate metabolism in the pregnant female. There is an increased tendency to ketosis.
   C. Insulin deficiency results in decreased protein synthesis and increased protein and fat catabolism.
   D. **Two types of diabetes mellitus**
      1. **Type I** is an insulin-dependent diabetes of juvenile onset and is associated with decreased insulin secretion.
      2. **Type II** is non-insulin-dependent diabetes. Serum insulin levels are low or normal. The tissues are essentially nonsensitive to insulin. Type II diabetes can develop in patients who are overweight.

III. **Clinical Findings:** Diagnosis is made on the basis

of two abnormal venous plasma glucose values on a 3-hour oral glucose tolerance test following a 100-mg oral glucose challenge. Two or more of the following values must be met or exceeded: fasting ≤105 mg/dL, 1 hour ≤190 mg/dL, 2 hour ≤165 mg/dL, 3 hour ≤145 mg/dL.

IV. Obstetric Management

A. The incidence of abortion is increased in the poorly controlled diabetic.

B. The incidence of polyhydramnios is increased.

C. The incidence of pre-eclampsia is increased.

D. The likelihood of an excessively large fetus is increased.

E. Dystocia and operative delivery are more frequent.

F. **Fetal effects** can include the following: fetal macrosomia, fetal death in utero, hydramnios, malpresentation, pre-eclampsia, and fetal malformation. Fetal death in utero occurs during the last 4 weeks of pregnancy. The perinatal mortality rate is 10 to 30%. Fetal hypoglycemia may be seen due to hyperplasia of the islets of Langerhans.

G. The patients are usually delivered between 36 and 38 weeks if the L/S ratio indicates pulmonary maturity. (L/S ratio 3·5 decreases incidence of RDS.)

H. The intravenous glucose tolerance test (GTT) gives the best results and aids in the diagnosis.

I. Modified White Classification

Class A: Diagnosis made on abnormal GTT

B: Onset after age 20, duration more than 10 years, with no vascular disease

C: Onset age 10 to 20, duration 10 to 19 years, vascular disease absent or minimal

D: Onset before age 10, duration more than 20 years, vascular disease present

E: Calcification of pelvic arteries

R: Proliferative retinopathy or vitreous hemorrhage

F: Nephropathy

RF: Criteria for classes R and F coexist

H: Arteriosclerotic heart disease evident

T: Prior renal transplant (the more advanced the disease, the worse the neonatal outcome)

J. Insulin is not always needed in all pregnant patients with type II diabetes. The objective of insulin therapy is to keep fasting plasma glucose levels between 60 and 100 mg/dL.

K. The insulin requirements are not predictable during pregnancy.

L. One should keep the blood sugar less than 120 mg/dL.

M. Infants born to diabetic mothers can be lethargic, edematous, and prone to atelectasis. One must keep this in mind if the neonate requires resuscitation.

N. Immediately postpartum, the diabetic mother may show a sharp decline in insulin requirements. Therefore, one should monitor the blood sugar frequently.

O. If **ketoacidosis** occurs, hydrate with 1/2 normal saline, give potassium if hypokalemia is present, and treat metabolic acidosis with sodium bicarbonate if the arterial pH is less than 7.1.

V. Anesthetic Considerations

  A. Increased susceptibility to aortocaval compression may be seen secondary to hydramnios.

  B. Patients are unusually sensitive to local anesthetic solutions.

  C. Dextrose 5% at 125 mL/hour should be infused during labor.

  D. One should check the blood sugar hourly.

  E. If the blood sugar is:

  1. 60 to 100 mg/dL: No action needs to be taken.

  2. Over 120 mg/dL: Continuous insulin infusion at 0.5 units/hour.

  3. If the blood sugar level falls, one should treat hypoglycemia with dextrose.

  F. The anesthetic goal is to avoid maternal hyperglycemia, fetal hyperglycemia in utero, and rebound hypoglycemia in neonatal period.

  G. Epidural anesthesia can be used for labor and delivery (avoid hypotension because decreased uteroplacental perfusion may exist).

  H. Either regional or general anesthesia may be done for cesarean section. If general anesthesia must be administered, one must be aware that diabetic patients may have large gastric volumes.

  I. Postoperatively, maternal insulin doses must be regulated carefully because maternal insulin requirements may change. The insulin requirement usually decreases.

J. Intraoperatively, a serum blood glucose should be done hourly.

SUGGESTED READING

Coustan DR. Recent advances in the management of diabetic pregnant women. *Clin Perinatol.* 1980; 7:299.

Jones CJP, Fox H. Placental changes in gestational diabetes: An ultrastructural study. *Obstet Gynecol.* 1976; 48:274.

Kitzmiller JL, Cloherty JP, Younger D, et al. Diabetic pregnancy and perinatal morbidity. *Am J Obstet Gynecol.* 1978; 131:560.

Soler NG, Malins JM. Diabetic pregnancy. Management of diabetes on the day of delivery. *Diabetologica.* 1978; 15:441.

27

Anesthetic Considerations for the Patient with Thyroid Disease

I. Incidence
    A. Thyroid function remains essentially normal during pregnancy. There is no increase in goiter during pregnancy as once thought.
    B. Hypothyroidism can be diagnosed by a low serum T4 level. The incidence is less than 4% in pregnant patients. Hypothyroid patients rarely become pregnant.
    C. Hyperthyroidism: The incidence is less than 2% of pregnancies.

II. General Considerations
    A. Hypothyroidism
        1. A slight thyroid deficiency may be noted in pregnant patients in general.
        2. Severe hypothyroidism may result in abortion, premature labor, and congenital fetal anomalies.
    B. Hyperthyroidism
        1. There is increased uptake of ingested radionuclide by the maternal thyroid gland, which suggests a hyperthyroid state.
        2. During pregnancy, there may be some enlargement of the thyroid gland caused by hyperplasia of thyroid gland tissue.

3. If **thyrotoxicosis** occurs, it can be serious for both the patient and fetus.

4. Thyrotoxicosis can increase the incidence of premature delivery and postpartum hemorrhage.

III. Clinical Findings for Hyperthyroidism

A. A serum total T4 greater than 15 μg/dL or a T3 greater than 220 ng/dL suggests hyperthyroidism.

B. A normal resin T3 uptake with an elevated T4 or T3 is diagnostic of hyperthyroidism.

IV. Obstetric Management

A. Hypothyroidism

1. Treatment: Thyroid supplement (levothyroxine, 160 to 200 ng daily) may be given or desiccated thyroid may be given during pregnancy.

2. Thyroid supplement overdosage can cause nervousness, tremors, tachycardia, sweating, vomiting, diarrhea, and weight loss.

3. These patients are sensitive to cardiovascular and CNS depressants (eg, general anesthetics, narcotics).

B. Hyperthyroidism

1. Treatment for hyperthyroidism is with propylthiouracil or methimazole.

2. If a **thyroid storm** occurs, immediate aggressive therapy is essential.

   a. Propylthiouracil, 150 to 200 mg q6h, may be administered to block thyroid hormone synthesis.

   b. Propranolol may be of benefit in the patient with thyrotoxicosis because it can effect catecholamine production. It may be given in 0.5-mg increments.

    c. Cortisol, 100 to 200 mg, should be given intravenously every 8 hours.

    d. Sodium iodide, 500 to 1000 mg, can be given intravenously to suppress secretion of the stored hormones.

    e. An intravenous infusion of **chilled crystalloid solution** containing glucose is indicated. Aggressive infusion of fluids may be necessary because of fluid loss secondary to hyperthermia.

    f. Because these patients can go into high output cardiac failure, invasive monitoring may become necessary.

    g. A high inspired oxygen concentration must also be given.

V. Anesthetic Considerations

  A. Hypothyroidism: Patients with hypothyroidism may have a history of paresthesias and hoarseness. These patients can be sensitive to inhalational anesthetics, as well as narcotics and benzodiazepines.

  B. Hyperthyroidism

    1. Tachycardia, elevated temperature, and increased blood pressure may occur under general anesthesia, making it difficult in assessing anesthesia depth.

    2. Either epidural or spinal anesthesia is preferred for cesarean section.

    3. Ketamine should be avoided in the patient with hyperthyroid disease.

    4. If ephedrine must be used to treat hypotension following regional anesthesia, it should be given intravenously in 2.5-mg increments.

SUGGESTED READING

Burrow GN. The management of thyrotoxicosis in pregnancy. *N Engl J Med*. 1982; 313:562.

Levy RP, Newman DM, Rejali LS, et al. The myth of goiter in pregnancy. *Am J Obstet Gynecol*. 1980; 137:701.

Mestman JH. Thyroid disease in pregnancy. *Clin Perinatol*. 1985; 12:3.

Stehling LC. Anesthetic management of the patient with hyperthyroidism. *Anesthesiology*. 1974; 41:585.

28

Anesthetic Considerations for the Pregnant Patient with Respiratory Disease

General Respiratory Physiology Changes During Pregnancy: Oxygen consumption increases 25% and minute ventilation 40%. Approximately 65% of healthy pregnant patients complain of dyspnea during the first 2 trimesters of pregnancy. Pulmonary embolization and asthma may on occasion be life threatening.

I. Pulmonary Embolus

    A. Pulmonary embolization is a dangerous complication of venous thrombosis. A cesarean section, a forceps delivery, and multiparity are situations related to an increased incidence of a pulmonary embolus.

    B. The pregnant patient is hypercoagulable. The pregnant patient may show increased susceptibility to deep vein thrombosis. The risk of an embolus is five times that of the non-pregnant female patient.

    C. Cesarean section patients are at a greater risk than those patients who had a vaginal delivery.

D. Pulmonary embolus is the leading cause of non-obstetric postpartum death.

E. Diagnosis: Tachypnea, dyspnea, anxiety, tachycardia, and chest pain may be noted. Right axis deviation may be noted on ECG. Jugular venous distention secondary to right ventricular failure. Dyspnea with lower extremity pain may be the only complaint.

F. Laboratory results

1. The ABG may reveal arterial hypoxemia. Alveolar dead space can be increased, which may be reflected in an elevated arterial carbon dioxide tension.

2. Chest x-rays may reveal an infiltrate or pleural effusion.

3. Pulmonary function testing can reveal increased dead space in the case of a pulmonary embolus.

4. If there is a question concerning the diagnosis, a lung scan can be useful.

5. Pulmonary arteriography is the definitive test for a pulmonary embolus.

G. Treatment

1. Oxygen must be administered. Maternal hypoxia may result in a dead or brain-damaged fetus. The patient may require intubation.

2. Heparin is administered intravenously (5000 units) followed by an infusion to maintain the PTT 2 to 2.5 times the control. Protamine sulfate (2 mg/l00 units of the hourly dose of heparin) will reverse heparin.

3. Heparin does not cross the placenta.

4. A hazard of heparin is **spontaneous hem-**

orrhage. Heparin should not be given to patients who have a bleeding problem or when the platelets are decreased since heparin can cause thrombocytopenia.

5. **Aminophylline** may be needed if the patient develops bronchospasm; 2 to 3 mg/kg can be infused over 20 minutes. An infusion of 0.5 mg/kg/hour may be used.

6. Cardiac ventricular arrhythmias usually respond to intravenous **lidocaine** (1 mg/kg).

7. **Isoproteronol** decreases pulmonary vascular resistance and may be useful if the cardiac output decreases (0.05 to 0.20 µg/kg/minute).

8. **Digitalis, dopamine,** and **dobutamine** may be helpful in maintaining the cardiac output, depending on the patient's hemodynamic status following pulmonary embolization (digitalis, 0.25 to 0.5 mg IV, dopamine, 2 to 10 µg/kg/minute, dobutamine, 2.5 to 10 µg/kg/minute).

9. **Coumarin** crosses the placenta and may cause fetal hemorrhage.

10. Coumarin may also be teratogenic.

11. The antidote to coumarin is 5 mg of intravenous vitamin K.

12. **Fresh frozen plasma** may also antagonize the effects of coumarin and should be used when rapid correction of coumarin anticoagulation is necessary.

13. Coumarin should not be used in a patient with a history of bleeding.

H. Anesthetic considerations

1. Regional anesthesia should not be used in anticoagulated patients.

   2. If a general anesthetic must be done for a cesarean section, ketamine (1 mg/kg) may be used for induction as hypotension should be avoided.
   3. Inhalational agents may be used.
   4. Nitrous oxide can be used unless evidence of increased pulmonary vascular resistance is evident.

II. Asthma

Asthma is a disease characterized by hyperreactive airways with increased airway secretions.

A. Incidence
   1. The incidence of asthma in pregnancy is approximately 1%.
   2. Pregnancy does not alter the course of the disease.
   3. Pregnant patients can worsen in the last trimester. Some patients, however, show improvement during the first trimester.

B. Fetal effects
   1. There can be a slight decrease in birth weight.
   2. With severe asthma, fetal mortality can be increased.
   3. Growth retardation is increased in the patient with severe asthma.

C. Treatment
   1. Management is the same as for nonpregnant patients.
   2. Xanthine bronchodilators and corticosteroids are not harmful to the fetus and may be used when necessary.
   3. Acute attack:
      a. Hypoxemia, acidosis, hypercarbia, and

    pulsus paradoxus greater than 10 torr require immediate treatment.

  b. Oxygen should be administered. The PaO_2 should be kept greater than 70 torr.

  c. Hydration should be restored.

  d. Aminophylline, 2 to 3 mg/kg, should be infused intravenously over 20 minutes. The maintenance infusion depends on the patient's aminophylline level. The therapeutic range is 10 to 20 μg/mL.

  e. Terbutaline, 0.25 mg, can be given subcutaneously if indicated.

  f. With a history of steroids, hydrocortisone 150 to 250 mg may be administered.

D. Anesthetic considerations

  1. Regional anesthesia is recommended for labor and delivery and a cesarean section if necessary.

  2. Ketamine is recommended over thiopental for induction of general anesthesia because of its beneficial effects on airway resistance if not contraindicated.

  3. The administration of 1 to 2 mg/kg of **lidocaine** administered intravenously before extubation of the trachea may prevent bronchospasm upon extubation.

  4. The endotracheal tube should not be removed until the patient has regained laryngeal and pharyngeal reflexes. A lidocaine infusion of 2 mg/kg/hour may be of benefit in attenuating airway stimulation until the patient can be extubated.

SUGGESTED READING

Bahna SL, Bjerkedal T. The course and outcome of pregnancy in women with bronchial asthma. *Acta Allergol.* 1972; 27:397.

Barber HRK. What is your most difficult problem? Anticoagulation during pregnancy. *Female Patient.* 1985; 10:71.

Bell WR, Royall RM. Heparin-associated thrombocytopenia: A comparison of three heparin preparations. *N Engl J Med.* 1980; 303:902.

Hernandez E, Angell CS, Johnson JWC. Asthma in pregnancy. *Curr Concepts Obstet Gynecol.* 1980; 55:739.

Laros RK, Alger LS. Thromboembolism and pregnancy. *Clin Obstet Gynecol.* 1979; 22:371.

Shnider SM, Papper EM. Anesthesia for the asthmatic patient. *Anesthesiology.* 1961; 22:886.

Villasanta U. Thromboembolic disease in pregnancy. *Am J Obstet Gynecol.* 1965; 93:142.

Weinberger SE, Weiss ST, Cohen WR, et al. Pregnancy and the lung. *Am Rev Respir Dis.* 1980; 121:559.

Weinstein AM, Dubin BD, Podleski WK, et al. Asthma and pregnancy. *JAMA.* 1979; 241:1161.

29

Anesthetic Considerations for the Patient with Cardiac Disease

Congenital heart disease is the principal heart problem complicating pregnancy. Pregnancy increases the cardiac output, the heart rate, and the blood volume, which all may worsen a myocardial condition. In most patients, changes in cardiovascular physiology during pregnancy do not have a significant effect on maternal or fetal well-being.

I. Incidence: The incidence is 1 to 2% in obstetric patients.

II. General Considerations
   A. Most lesions are rheumatic in origin (88.2%).
   B. Congenital lesions account for approximately 11.7% of the lesions.
   C. Myocarditis, thyrotoxic heart disease and advanced hypertensive heart disease are extremely rare.
   D. The principal hazard of heart disease in the pregnant patient is congestive heart failure.
   E. With marked pathology, maternal mortality is 1 to 3%.
   F. New York Heart Association Classification
      1. I. Disease with no limitation of physical activity.

2. II. Disease with slight limitation of physical activity.

3. III. Disease with marked limitation of physical activity. Comfortable at rest; less than ordinary activity causes symptoms.

4. IV. Disease with symptoms even at rest (symptoms: cough following exertion, palpitations, edema, shortness of breath).

5. The higher the classification, the higher the incidence of congestive heart failure.

6. The most common lesion involves the mitral valve.

7. The functional capacity of the heart is the best single measurement of cardiac status.

III. Clinical Findings
A. Mitral or aortic valvular disease

1. One should put the patient on her left side for auscultation of the mitral lesion.

2. With mitral stenosis, a low-pitched mid-diastolic murmur may be auscultated.

3. With mitral regurgitation, a pansystolic murmur can be heard.

4. Aortic insufficiency may be found alone in 10% of pregnant women with heart disease or it may be accompanied by a mitral lesion in 10% of pregnant women.

5. One should have the patient lean forward and expire during auscultation.

6. One should auscultate the left third or fourth intercostal space at the lower end of the sternum.

7. A soft blowing diastolic murmur at the right third intercostal space suggests aortic insufficiency.

8. Rheumatic mitral stenosis is the most important cardiac lesion of clinical significance during pregnancy.

9. Death

    a. Fifty percent of deaths occur in patients with valvular heart disease within 24 hours of delivery.

    b. One third occur within the next 4 days.

    c. Death is due to one of the following:

        (1) Pulmonary edema and congestive heart failure (75%)

        (2) Bacterial endocarditis (15%)

        (3) Peritonitis (49%)

10. Obstetric management

    a. Strenuous effort on the part of the patient (ie, bearing down) should be avoided.

    b. Mortality can be increased 2 to 3 times with vaginal delivery in patients with severe heart disease. A cesarean section may be of more benefit to the patient with a class III or IV lesion.

B. Mitral stenosis

    1. During labor and vaginal delivery, if an epidural anesthetic is administered, an epidural dose must be given slowly to prevent a decrease in SVR.

    2. Hypotension should be treated with fluids and metaraminol (10 mg/250 mg saline).

    3. With severe mitral stenosis, a slow induction with halothane with cricoid pressure can be done if an emergency cesarean section must be done.

4. Hypovolemia is not tolerated well.

C. Mitral regurgitation

1. The myocardium must not be depressed by an anesthetic.

2. Regional anesthesia for vaginal delivery is recommended.

3. For cesarean section, regional anesthesia is recommended as one should prevent increases in the SVR.

D. Aortic insufficiency

1. Regional anesthesia is recommended to decrease SVR.

2. If heart failure is present, do not depress heart further if a general anesthetic must be administered. Therefore, avoid N_2O.

E. Aortic stenosis

1. Labor pain is best managed with systemic medication.

2. High dose fentanyl can be used for general anesthesia.

3. If an epidural is to be done, one must dose it slowly to avoid decreases in SVR. Bupivacaine may be the agent of choice because of its slower onset.

F. Congenital heart disease

1. Atrial septal defect (ASD) and **ventricular septal defects** (VSD) are common. When doing an epidural block, one must avoid a decrease in SVR, which could reverse a left-to-right shunt (L-R).

2. Atrial septal defect:

a. Supraventricular arrhythmias can increase a L-R shunt.

    b. An increase in the SVR can increase a L-R shunt.

    c. A decrease in the pulmonary vascular resistance (PVR) can increase a L-R shunt.

    d. PVR increases with hypoxia and hypercarbia.

  3. VSD

    a. An increase in SVR can increase a L-R shunt.

    b. An increase in the heart rate increases the L-R shunt.

    c. A PVR increase exacerbates pulmonary hypertension.

  4. A pulmonary artery catheter can go through the defect, therefore, erroneous readings may be obtained.

G. With a **patent ductus arteriosus,** epidural anesthesia/analgesia can be used for labor or cesarean section.

H. Tetralogy of Fallot

  1. A decrease in SVR increases L-R shunt.

  2. Segmental epidural anesthesia for labor (T10-T12) may be done.

  3. General anesthesia for cesarean section is recommended.

  4. Arterial line and central venous pressure monitoring should be done as part of the anesthetic management.

I. Eisenmenger's syndrome

  1. Severe pulmonary hypertension secondary to prolonged ASD or VSD may be seen.

  2. Sudden death can occur during parturition and during the puerperium.

3. A decrease in SVR can increase a R-L shunt.

4. A decrease in blood volume decreases pulmonary blood flow.

5. An increase in the PVR increases a R-L shunt.

6. Pulmonary artery catheters may not be advisable in these patients.

7. Arterial line and central venous pressure monitoring should be done.

J. Hypertrophic cardiomyopathy

1. The intravascular volume must be maintained.

2. The SVR should be increased.

3. A decrease in contractility of the heart is desirable.

4. One must avoid regional for labor.

5. General anesthesia for cesarean section (avoid cardiovascular stimulation) should be done.

6. To decrease the outflow gradient, beta antagonists, myocardial depressants, hypervolemia, and peripheral vasoconstrictors may all be used.

K. Cardiomyopathy of pregnancy

1. Cardiomyopathy occurs during pregnancy or the first 6 months postpartum.

2. One may do epidural anesthesia/analgesia for labor or cesarean section.

3. With severe ventricular failure, a slow narcotic induction with cricoid pressure should be done to induce general anesthesia. Postpartum cardiomyopathy is a disorder of heart muscle and is probably viral in origin. Low output cardiac failure may be seen.

L. Primary pulmonary hypertension

1. Death during labor and puerperium has been reported.
2. Hypercarbia, hypoxia, acidosis, high pulmonary inflation pressures all increase pulmonary vascular resistance.
3. A decrease in venous return causes a fall in right and left ventricular output.
4. A decrease in SVR can cause cardiac decompensation.
5. Right ventricular dysfunction is exacerbated by myocardial depressants.
6. An arterial line and pulmonary catheter should be inserted before an anesthetic.
7. General anesthesia must be done for cesarean section.
8. A deep level of anesthesia before intubation is desirable.
9. If an epidural is placed for labor, it must be dosed slowly.

SUMMARY OF VALVULAR AND CONGENITAL DISEASE

	HEART RATE	PRE-LOAD	CONTRACT-ILITY	AFTER-LOAD
Aortic stenosis	Avoid bradycardia and marked tachycardia	Maintain with fluids	Prevent decreases	Avoid decreases in the SVR
Aortic insufficiency	Avoid bradycardia; maintain the heart rate	Maintain with fluids	Prevent decreases	Avoid increases in the SVR

SUMMARY

	HEART RATE	PRE-LOAD	CONTRACT-ILITY	AFTER-LOAD
	between 80–100 bpm			
Mitral stenosis	Avoid tachycardia	Maintain with fluids	Maintain	Avoid decreases in the SVR
Mitral insufficiency	Avoid bradycardia	Maintain	Maintain	Avoid increases in the SVR
Congestive heart failure	Avoid bradycardia	Maintain	Maintain	Avoid increases in the SVR

Invasive monitoring should be used in patients with moderate-to-severe signs and symptoms. Signs suggestive of underlying cardiac disease include a diastolic murmur, cyanosis, clubbing, a systolic flow murmur, and jugular venous distention.

IV. Obstetric Management
   A. Appropriate evaluation by a cardiologist when signs and symptoms indicate.
   B. Counseling and education to attenuate anxiety.
   C. Antiobiotic prophylaxis in patients with a history of rheumatic fever or prosthetic heart valve. (Ampicillin, 2 g IV or IM and gentamycin, 1.5 mg/kg IV or IM 1 hour before delivery and 8 hours postpartum. Vancomycin, 1 g can be given instead of ampicillin if the patient is allergic to penicillin.)
V. Anesthetic Considerations: The choice of anesthetic depends on the patient's hemodynamic profile. A team approach with the obstetrician and

cardiologist will help one plan the most appropriate anesthetic.

SUGGESTED READING

Clark SL, Phelan JP, Greenspoon J, et al. Labor and delivery in the presence of mitral stenosis. Central hemodynamic observations. *Am J Obstet Gynecol.* 1985; 152:984.

Copeland WE, Wooley CF, Ryan JM, et al. Pregnancy and congenital heart disease. *Am J Obstet Gynecol.* 1963; 86:107.

Robinson S. Pulmonary artery catheters in Eisenmenger's Syndrome: Many risks, few benefits. *Anesthesiology* 1983; 58:588.

Shnider SM, Levinson G. Anesthesia for Obstetrics. Baltimore: Williams & Wilkins; 1987: 345.

Ueland K. Pregnancy and cardiovascular disease. *Med Clin North Am.* 1977; 61:17.

30

Anesthetic Considerations for the Pregnant Patient with Renal Disease

I. Incidence: The incidence of renal disease during pregnancy can be approximately 1 to 2%.

II. General Considerations

    A. During pregnancy, in most patients, renal blood flow increases. At 32 weeks' gestation, it rises by approximately 40%. The glomerular filtration rate (GFR) also increases during pregnancy. The upper normal limits of the serum creatinine is 0.58 mg/dL while the BUN is 9 mg/dL. There is an increased incidence of cystitis and pyelonephritis in pregnancy, which may be related to dilatation of the ureters, because the enlarged uterus can compress the ureters at the pelvic brim. Consequently, urinary tract infections are common during pregnancy. Pyelonephritis can occur during pregnancy. Patients may be hospitalized for the administration of antibiotics; because, if pyelonephritis is left untreated, it could progress to septic shock. Poststreptococcal glomerulonephritis can also occur during pregnancy, and these patients may develop superimposed pre-eclampsia or hypertension.

During pregnancy, acute renal failure, however, is rarely seen.

B. Hypertension. The parturient with severe renal disease may be hypertensive. **Hydralazine** can be used to treat hypertension and must be titrated slowly, because patients with renal disease may be sensitive to the vasodilatation caused by hydralazine in the presence of a depleted intravascular volume.

C. Monitoring. In parturients with mild kidney impairment, only routine monitoring is necessary. Depending on the severity of the renal failure, either central venous pressure (CVP) monitoring or pulmonary artery catheter monitoring may be indicated. If pulmonary artery catheter monitoring is indicated, then one should also consider the placement of an arterial line. The patient's overall medical condition should indicate what type of monitoring is necessary. The patient with cardiovascular compromise should be monitored with a pulmonary artery catheter and an arterial line.

D. Renal transplantation (postoperative). Menstruation resumes 1 to 12 months after successful surgery. Consequently, reproductive function is markedly improved. It should be noted that patients following renal transplantation will be taking immunosuppressive drugs; and, therefore, regional anesthesia must be administered with strict adherence to sterile technique.

III. Clinical Findings

Gestation has no effect on underlying **renal disease**. Proteinuria is not considered abnormal until urinary protein levels exceed 300 mg/24 hours.

Preanesthetic BUN and serum creatinine measurements should be done before administration of an anesthetic, and may be all that is needed for the parturient with minor renal impairment. In the presence of severe renal impairment, however, a creatinine clearance test should be done as it reflects the overall elimination ability of substances by the kidneys. Preanesthetic laboratory tests that may be useful are the following: A complete blood count, a bleeding time as well as the prothrombin (PT) and partial thromboplastin time (PTT), BUN, serum creatinine, a creatinine clearance when indicated, serum electrolytes, and a routine urinalysis. When indicated, one should obtain the following: liver function tests, an ECG, and ABG.

IV. Obstetric Management. Pregnant patients with severe renal disease may have a higher incidence of fetal death, preterm delivery, and intrauterine growth retardation than healthy parturients.

V. Anesthetic Considerations. The anesthetic management should be essentially the same as with any nonpregnant patient who has renal disease. It should be remembered that some changes in renal physiology could alter drug metabolism as well as excretion.

  A. General approach to anesthetic management. Before choosing an anesthetic technique, one should assess the history, physical examination, and laboratory values, and discuss the anesthetic options with the patients.

   1. Subarachnoid anesthesia. If a subarachnoid block is considered, one must estimate the patient's plasma volume by a careful history, physical examination, and laboratory analysis. In the patient with only mild renal impairment, a subarachnoid block can be used. In a patient with moderate-to-severe hypertension with a depleted plasma volume, however, one should consider epidural for vaginal delivery, or general anesthesia for cesarean section.

2. **Epidural anesthesia.** If epidural anesthesia is used for labor pain or for cesarean section, it should be dosed slowly, preferably with a local anesthetic that has a slow onset (ie, bupivacaine). Furthermore, one must redose the epidural catheter slowly (1 mL/minute) to minimize the incidence of hypotension.

3. **General anesthesia.** If general anesthesia is considered, ethrane should be avoided, because of its potential for fluoride nephrotoxicity. During the induction of general anesthesia, the parturients with renal disease may respond as if they are hypovolemic and become hypotensive. Etomidate (0.3 mg/kg) might be considered instead of thiopental for the induction of general anesthesia. For the first and second stages of labor, epidural analgesia minimizes the stress and catecholamine release caused by labor pain. It should be remembered that the liver metabolizes amide local anesthetics and, when used in minimal concentrations, the volumes of distribution and clearance rates remain unaltered. Furthermore, ester local anesthetics undergo hydrolysis by plasma cho-

linesterase, which are not affected in patients with renal disease.

a. Fentanyl. Fentanyl may be used with bupivacaine during labor and for the maintenance of general anesthesia after delivery of the baby, because it undergoes non-renal elimination.

b. Hyperkalemia. Increase in serum potassium may be noted following **succinylcholine administration** in patients with renal disease. If the serum potassium is 5 mEq^0 or greater, succinylcholine should not be used during the induction of general anesthesia. Atracurium, 0.4 to 0.5 mg/kg may be used or 0.08 to 0.10 mg/kg of vercuronium may be considered as alternatives to succinylcholine. Either of these muscle relaxants may be used interoperatively and the choice depends on the anticipated duration of surgery.

c. Succinylcholine. Occasionally, a prolonged response to succinylcholine might be noted secondary to a decreased cholinesterase activity. Consequently, a nerve stimulator should be used during general anesthesia and muscle relaxants should be titrated to effect using a nerve stimulator.

d. Transfusions. Packed red cells should be used to replace significant blood loss interoperatively as needed.

e. Hypertension. The parturient with renal disease should be closely monitored, not only interoperatively, but also in the postoperative recovery area, for the incidence of hypertension. Either nitroprusside or hydralazine may be used to treat hypertension perioperatively.

4. Coagulopathies. Coagulopathies may exist in the parturient with renal disease and must be taken into consideration before attempting any regional anesthetic. In most instances, a regional anesthetic is preferred over a general anesthetic, unless the patient has a coagulopathy. Furthermore, decreased platelet adhesiveness may be noted, which may be manifested as a prolonged bleeding time.

SUGGESTED READING

Bear RA. Pregnancy in patients with renal disease: A study of 44 cases. *Obstet Gynecol.* 1976; 48:13.

Davison JM, Lindatimer MD. Renal disease in pregnant women. *Clin Obstet Gynecol.* 1978; 21:411.

Duff P. Pyelonephritis in pregnant patients. *Clin Obstet Gynecol.* 1984; 27:17.

Madden PJ. Anesthesia for the patient with impaired renal function. *Anesth Intensive Care.* 1983; 11:321.

Miller RD, Gianfaga W, Ackerly JA, et al. Succinylcholine-induced hyperkalemia in patients with renal failure. *Anesthesiology.* 1972; 36:138.

Waltzer WC, et al. Pregnancy in renal transplantation. *Transplant Proc.* 1980; 12:221.

31

Anesthetic Considerations for the Morbidly Obese Patient

I. Incidence. Six percent of pregnant patients are obese, while 1 to 2% are morbidly obese.

II. General Considerations

A. Surgery and pregnancy pose significant hazards to the morbidly obese woman. An ideal weight (kg) = height (cm) − 100.

B. Total fetal growth is primarily influenced by the quantity of maternal body stores and fetal growth is influenced less by maternal caloric intake.

C. An excessive weight gain or pre-existing obesity can be associated with increased fetal and maternal morbidity. A normal weight gain is 20 to 30 lb during pregnancy.

D. Individuals in excess of 20% of the ideal body weight for height are obese. Morbid obesity is a body weight twice normal.

E. Complications related to obesity include:

  1. Large babies

  2. Breech presentation

  3. Hypertension

  4. Diabetes

III. Clinical Findings

A. A decrease in functional residual capacity may

be seen that is more than the non-obese pregnant female.
B. Cardiac output increases significantly.
C. The systolic and diastolic blood pressures may
be elevated.
D. Cardiac work and myocardial oxygen consumption are increased.
E. Delayed gastric emptying can occur in addition
to hyperacidity and diminished lower esophageal sphincter tone.
F. An increased gastric volume may be present.
IV. Obstetric Management. Massive obesity may be
associated with prolonged labor and abnormal fetal presentation, which may result in the need for
a cesarean section in some patients.
V. Anesthetic Considerations
  A. Epidural analgesia decreases respiratory work
  and oxygen consumption.
  B. Oxygen should be administered throughout labor because of increased oxygen consumption.
  C. Technical difficulties may be encountered when
  performing regional anesthesia because of fat
  over the spinous processes. Special long
  needles may be necessary.
  D. The sitting position may provide the anesthetist with the easiest identification of the midline.
  E. The volume of anesthetic needed for spinal anesthesia may be less. It is controversial
  whether or not decreased volume is needed
  for epidural anesthesia.
  F. Aortocaval compression must be avoided.
  G. Histamine H_2-receptor antagonists should be
  administered before surgery.
  H. Metoclopramide (10 mg IV) may be of benefit.

I. All patients should receive 30 mL of 0.3 M sodium citrate.

J. Obese patients can have laryngeal edema. Therefore, a smaller diameter (6.5 mm) endo-tracheal tube should be prepared if general anesthesia is anticipated.

K. A short-handled laryngoscope blade may make intubation easier if general anesthesia is necessary.

L. Postoperative analgesia is helpful to encourage deep breathing as well as atelectasis. Epidural narcotics may be administered.

M. A massive panniculus can make intubation potentially difficult. One may tape the panniculus to the ether screen.

SUGGESTED READING

Blass NH. Regional anesthesia in the morbidly obese. *Reg Anesth.* 1979; 4:26.

Eng M, Butler J, Bonica J. Respiratory function in pregnant obese women. *Am J Obstet Gynecol.* 1975; 123:241.

Freedman MA, Wilds PL, George WM, et al. Grotesque obesity: A serious complication of labor and delivery. *South Med J.* 1972; 65:732.

32

Anesthetic Considerations for the Patient with Disseminated Intravascular Coagulation (DIC)

I. **Incidence.** Disseminated intravascular coagulation can exceed an incidence of 25% in parturients with death in utero greater than 4 weeks.

II. **General Considerations**
   A. During pregnancy, DIC occurs secondary to another disease process.
   B. DIC is mediated by activation of thrombi leading to the production of fibrin, consumption of clotting factors, diminution of platelets, and activation of the fibrinolytic systems.
   C. The patient who survives the acute bleeding can die from ischemic damage to the lungs or kidneys.
   D. **Etiology.** Causes of DIC include shock; infection, including bacterial, rickettsial, viral, fungal, and parasitic; abruptio placenta; amniotic fluid embolism; intrauterine fetal death; and pre-eclampsia-eclampsia.

III. **Clinical Findings**
   A. Thrombocytopenia is present due to widely disseminated clotting, which consumes platelets and results in a prolonged bleeding time.

    B. Factors I, II, V, and VIII are decreased. As a result, patients will exhibit a prolonged PT and activated PTT.

    C. Fibrin degradation products will be present in the plasma.

    D. A prolonged thrombin time will be present.

    E. Fibrinogen levels will be markedly decreased.

IV. Obstetric Management

    A. One should treat the underlying etiology of DIC.

    B. Ideally, the coagulation defect should be corrected before surgery.

    C. The transfusion of platelets is necessary.

    D. Fresh frozen plasma should be administered if the patient is bleeding severely (2 to 3 units).

    E. If serious bleeding continues, cryoprecipitate may be given.

    F. The mere establishment of a diagnosis of DIC is not cause to treat. One should observe for signs of frank bleeding from tissues.

    G. Acidosis should be treated with sodium bicarbonate.

    H. The use of heparin and epsilon-aminocaproic acid is controversial.

    I. One should maintain adequate tissue perfusion.

    J. After each blood volume exchange (approximately 5 liters), give 6 units of plasma.

    K. After a 10-liter blood volume exchange, give 6 more units of plasma, 5 units of platelets, and 10 units of cryoprecipitate.

V. Anesthetic Considerations

    A. Large bore intravenous lines (2) should be established for volume replacement.

B. Arterial line placement should be considered.
C. CVP or pulmonary artery catheter monitoring, or both, may be helpful in the management of the restoration of volume replacement. Invasive monitoring should be done when the clotting abnormalities have been corrected.
D. For general anesthesia, ketamine, 1 mg/kg, should be used for induction.
E. If an epidural catheter was placed before the onset of DIC, one should have a normal PT, PTT, and bleeding time before removing the epidural catheter.

SUGGESTED READING

Ebner H. The obstetric anesthesiologist: His role in coagulation disorders in the parturient. *Anesth Analg*. 1971; 50:131.

Heene DL. Disseminated intravascular coagulation: Evaluation of therapeutic approaches. *Semin Throb Hemostas*. 1977; 4:291.

Kleiner GJ, Mersey C, Johnson AJ, et al. Defibrination in normal and abnormal parturition. *Br J Haematol*. 1970; 19:159.

Redman CW. Coagulation problems in human pregnancy. *Postgrad Med J*. 1979; 55:367.

33

Anesthetic Considerations for the Patient with Sickle Cell Disease

I. Incidence
   A. Sickle cell disease is caused by inheritance of a gene for sickle cell hemoglobin (S). When hemoglobin S genes are inherited from both parents (SS), severe anemia and bone pain may occur. With one hemoglobin S gene, a less severe anemia occurs.
   B. The incidence of sickle cell trait is 8 to 9/100 black Americans. The incidence of homozygous sickle cell disease is 1/625 American blacks.

II. General Considerations
   A. Sickle cell hemoglobinopathies exhibit autosomal dominant inheritance.
   B. Sickle cell disease can be associated with increased fetal death.
   C. Patients with double heterozygous sickle cell disease may not have problems until the last trimester of pregnancy.
   D. Patients with homozygous disease have repeated sickle cell crises not only in pregnancy but throughout life.
   E. Antepartum problems are rarely seen.
   F. These patients are susceptible to anoxia.

G. Pregnancy does not subject these patients to additional risks.

III. Clinical Findings

A. If target cells, reticulocytes or sickle cells are noted, a screening test for sickle cell hemoglobin should be done.

B. Megablastic anemia may be appreciated in parturients with sickle cell anemia.

IV. Obstetric Management

A. Maternal risks

1. Sickle cell crises

2. Infection

3. Cardiac and pulmonary complications (congestive heart failure and marrow embolization)

B. Fetal risks

1. Fetal miscarriage and stillbirths are increased.

2. The fetal death rate can be high.

C. Treatment

1. It is controversial as to whether or not partial exchange transfusions with red blood cells containing normal hemoglobin should be started at the end of the second trimester and repeated every 2 weeks to keep the hematocrit greater than 40% in patients with sickle cell disease.

2. Fetal monitoring should be done during exchange transfusion.

3. If a crisis occurs, an exchange transfusion is required.

4. Oxygen should be administered in the presence of a crisis.

5. The patient must be hydrated and kept comfortable and warm.

6. Infections must be treated. Urine should be cultured frequently if infection is suspected.
7. Acidosis must be corrected.
8. An adequate blood volume must be maintained with adequate replacement when needed.

V. Anesthetic Considerations

A. Regional anesthesia can be used only with caution in the untransfused patient with sickle cell anemia.
B. When regional anesthesia is administered, hypotension must be avoided.
C. One must be aware that spinal artery thrombosis can occur in the patient with sickle cell disease. This could possibly result in an anterior spinal artery syndrome.
D. During labor, the parturient with sickle cell disease must not be oversedated because of the potential for hypoxia and increased sickling. Consequently, one should use epidural or intraspinal narcotics only with extreme caution.

SUGGESTED READING

Charache S, Scott F, Niebyl J, et al. Management of sickle cell disease in pregnant patients. *Obstet Gynecol*. 1980; 55:407.

Ferguson JE, O'Reilly RA. Hemoglobin E and pregnancy. *Obstet Gynecol*. 1985; 66:136.

Morrison JC, Blake PG, Reed CD, et al. Therapy for the pregnant patient with sickle hemoglobinopathies: A national focus. *Am J Obstet Gynecol*. 1982; 144:268.

Pastorek J. Maternal death associated with sickle cell trait. *Am J Obstet Gynecol*. 1985; 151:295.

34

Anesthetic Considerations for the Patient with Acquired Immune Deficiency Syndrome (AIDS)

I. Incidence. The incidence of AIDS in the parturient is not exactly known. A significant number of the 2 million adults in the United States infected with AIDS, however, is reported.

II. General Considerations

A. AIDS may be diagnosed in patients who develop malignancies or opportunistic infections because of suppression in cell-mediated immunity.

B. AIDS is the manifestation of opportunistic infections and malignancies caused by depression of the immune system. Both T and B lymphocytes are depressed.

C. The etiology of AIDS is the **human immunodeficiency virus (HIV),** which infects and destroys T lymphocytes.

D. HIV is found in blood, vaginal secretions, and semen. Other fluids that contain lymphocytes, such as saliva or cerebrospinal fluid, have not been found to transmit AIDS to date.

E. Ten percent of adults with AIDS are women.

Intravenous drug users comprise approximately 50% of females that have AIDS.

F. AIDS can be passed from the mother to the fetus.

G. AIDS can also be transmitted by heterosexual contact.

III. Clinical Findings

A. Pneumonia secondary to *Pneumocystis carinii* is not uncommon.

B. Kaposi's sarcoma can also occur as can herpes simplex infections.

C. **Symptoms** include fatigue, weight loss, diarrhea, anemia, fever, and thrombocytopenia.

D. The incubation period for AIDS can be 7 years or longer.

E. The **Western blot test** is a sensitive test for the detection of HIV antibodies.

F. Death is usually from sepsis or tumor growth.

IV. Obstetric Considerations.
Comprehensive management of the parturient with AIDS includes clinical and psychosocial care in the antepartum, intrapartum, and postpartum periods. All obstetric and neonatal health care personnel must protect themselves from exposure to HIV.

V. Anesthetic Managament

A. Gloves, masks, and protective eyewear must be worn during the anesthetic management.

B. One should not attempt to recap needles because of the potential for an accidental needle stick.

C. Disposable anesthetic circuits, ventilators, bellows, and soda lime canisters may be advisable.

D. The precise anesthetic management should be influenced by the manifestation of the disease.

E. Because of the chance for infection (due to a depressed immune system) and bleeding, placement of an epidural catheter may not be advisable in many instances.

F. Because of the potential risk of meningitis, a subarachnoid block may also not be advisable.

G. Pneumonia may make oxygenation of the patient difficult and, consequently, positive end-expiratory pressure (PEEP) may be needed intraoperatively.

H. Intravascular catheters and endotracheal tubes should be placed in such a manner as to avoid bacterial contaminations.

I. If an anesthetist experiences an accidental needle stick, serological testing must be initiated and repeated every 6 weeks to determine if transmission of the virus has occurred. It usually takes 6 to 12 weeks before a positive test is noted.

SUGGESTED READING

Curran JW, Lawrence DH, Jaffee H, et al. Acquired immunodeficiency syndrome (AIDS) associated with transfusions. *N Engl J Med.* 1984; 310:69.

Hedrion R. Pregnancy and AIDS. *Hum Reprod.* 1988; 3:257.

Ho DD, Pomerantz RJ, Kaplan J, et al. Pathogenesis of infection with human immunodeficiency virus. *N Engl J Med.* 1987; 317:278.

Kunkel SE, Warner MA. Human T cell lymphotrophic virus type III (HTLV-III) infection. How it can affect you, your patients and your anesthetic practice. *Anesthesiology*. 1987; 66:195.

Minkoff HL, Feinkindl L. Management of pregnancies of HIV-infected women. *Clin Obstet Gynecol*. 1989; 32:467.

Update. Acquired immunodeficiency syndrome—United States. *JAMA*. 1986; 257:433.

SECTION VIII

Special Considerations

35

Anesthetic Considerations for the Pregnant Substance Abuser

I. Incidence. A large portion of the substance-abusing population is of childbearing age. The incidence is difficult to determine because not all substance abusers admit their abuse.

II. General Considerations

  A. Substance abuse is the self-administration of non-prescribed drugs.

  B. Substance abuse can complicate both pregnancy and the management of anesthesia. Patients may be chronically dependent on drugs or be drug free at the time of admission.

  C. Drug addicts and their babies may develop tolerance to drugs, which may be manifested by an increased rate of hepatic metabolism or less maternal regressive receptors to anesthetic drugs.

III. Clinical Findings

  A. Drug withdrawal can occur and if it occurs preoperatively could be life threatening. Fetal drug withdrawal can also be life threatening.

  B. Withdrawal symptoms include the following: tachycardia, hypertension, diaphoresis, tremors, hyperthermia, metabolic acidosis, and ultimately the possibility of cardiovascular collapse. Withdrawal from meperidine can occur in 2 hours while methadone can take up to 48 hours.

C. Cocaine abuse in pregnant patients is associated with abruptio placenta.

D. Death from cocaine may be due to cardiac dysrhythmias. Seizures may occur in patients who abuse cocaine. Consequently, patients may present as eclamptic patients. Myocardial infarction and cerebrovascular accidents have also been reported. Because these patients may be hypertensive and have increased reflexes, the pregnant patient who abuses cocaine can present as a preeclamptic patient. Acute CNS stimulation is seen while chronically catecholamines are decreased.

E. Infant intoxication or fetal withdrawal can be noticed in the neonate following prolonged maternal drug exposure.

IV. Obstetric Management. Pregnant substance abusers may on occasion suffer from poor nutrition, hepatitis, abscesses, thrombophlebitis, and pulmonary embolus.

V. Anesthetic Considerations

A. Orthostatic hypotension can occur in the chronic substance abuser and can place the obstetric patient at an increased risk following regional anesthesia administration.

B. These patients may be enzyme induced. Consequently, during general anesthesia, these patients may require more anesthesia.

C. Intravenous access is usually difficult.

D. Pulmonary edema has been reported to occur in patients who abuse drugs.

E. AIDS may be a complication of parenteral drug abuse.

F. Hepatitis may be noted following parenteral drug abuse.

G. Infants of drug abusers can have apnea. This should be a consideration if one contemplates epidural opioids.

H. Epidural opioids (both agonist and agonist-antagonist) can cause withdrawal symptoms in these patients.

I. There may be alterations in infant neurobehavioral scores.

J. The sympathetic nervous system augmentation that occurs in the patient undergoing withdrawal can decrease uterine blood flow, consequently placing the fetus at risk.

K. Controlled methadone use has minimal effect or anesthetic requirements.

L. Uterine hyperactivity may be noted during narcotic withdrawal, which may decrease blood flow to the fetus.

M. The anesthetic of choice for either vaginal delivery or cesarean section in the acutely intoxicated patient depends upon the degree of intoxication and the interaction with the anesthetic technique or agent.

N. Substances abused

CATEGORY	AGENTS	ANESTHETIC IMPLICATIONS
CNS depressants	Ethanol Sedatives	Alcohol intoxication may decrease cytochrome P450

(continued)

CATEGORY	AGENTS	ANESTHETIC IMPLICATIONS
	Barbiturates Marijuana	enzyme function (local anesthetic metabolism may be affected). Withdrawal may occur. Tolerance to the CNS depressant effects of anesthetics following barbiturate abuse can occur. The newborn may be depressed.
CNS stimulants	Cocaine Amphet-amines	Acute use of these drugs can inhibit reuptake of catecholamines. Increased blood pressure and uterine tone may be seen. Beta-blocking agents can be used to treat tachycardia but unopposed alpha-adrenergic stimulation can produce severe hypertension.
Opiates	Narcotics	Narcotic abuse can result in premature birth. ACTH suppression can occur. Naloxone infusion reverses coma and hypotension following overdose. Clonidine may be harmful to the fetus. Methadone is safer.

The patient's overall medical condition should dictate the anesthetic plans. One should use AIDS precautions when treating the narcotic and cocaine abusers.

SUGGESTED READING

Barash P, Kopriva CJ, Langou R, et al. Is cocaine a sympathetic stimulant during general anesthesia? *JAMA.* 1980; 243:1437.

Cregler LL, Mark H. Medical complications of cocaine abuse. *N Engl J Med.* 1986; 315:1495.

Kenepp N, James FM, Wheeler AS. Substance abuse. In *Obstetric Anesthesia: The Complicated Patient.* Philadelphia: FA Davis; 1988: 505–530.

Martin JC. Irreversible changes in mature and aging animals following intrauterine drug exposure. *Neurobehav Toxicol Teratol.* 1986; 8:335.

Ramoska E, Sacchetti AD. Propranolol-induced hypertension in treatment of cocaine intoxication. *Ann Emerg Med.* 1985; 14:1112.

Stoelting RK, Dierdorf SF, McCammon RL, et al. Anesthesia and Co-Existing Disease. New York: Churchill-Livingstone; 1988: 729–747.

36

Anesthetic Considerations for the Patient with a Hydatidiform Mole-Molar Pregnancy

I. Incidence. Its incidence is 1/40,000 pregnancies and usually occurs during the first 18 weeks.

II. General Considerations

    A. Hydatidiform mole is a degenerative disorder of the chorion of unknown etiology.

    B. It is more common among women under age 20 and over age 40.

    C. It is more prevalent in Oriental females.

    D. The incidence is 1/1500 pregnancies.

    E. 80% of pregnancies are usually uncomplicated.

    F. When complications occur, they can be life threatening.

    G. Complications associated with molar pregnancy include the following:

        1. Pregnancy-induced hypertension

        2. Trophoblastic embolization

        3. Electrolyte abnormalities from persistent vomiting

        4. A hyperthyroid-like state with high output

cardiac failure (seen in patients with high human chorionic gonadotropin [hCG] levels)
5. Pulmonary edema
6. Severe bleeding
H. The incidence of malignancy is 4%.

III. Clinical Findings
A. Excessive nausea and vomiting may be noted.
B. Uterine bleeding may be noted.
C. The uterus is larger than expected.
D. A 24-hour urine hCG usually exceeds 500,000 IU/24 hours.
E. An elevated beta subunit of hCG is usually noted.

IV. Obstetric Management
A. The diagnosis is made by ultrasound.
B. Once the diagnosis is confirmed, evacuation of the molar pregnancy is indicated.
C. Suction curettage is the method of choice for evacuation.

V. Anesthetic Considerations
A. One must maintain hemodynamic stability during induction of general anesthesia.
B. One must minimize further bleeding (use a nitrous oxide/short-acting narcotic technique) instead of an inhalational agent.
C. One should keep the anesthetic depth deep because the possibility of an existing hyperthyroid state exists, which could result in tachycardia and hypertension.
D. Do not induce the patient with ketamine if the patient is hypovolemic because of the potential for marked tachycardia if a hyperthyroid state exists.
E. **Etomidate** (0.3 mg/kg) may be used for induction with unstable hemodynamics.

F. One should have **edrophonium,** 5 to 10 mg, or **phenylephrine,** 100 μg/mL, or **propranolol** (given in 0.5-mg increments) in syringes ready to treat tachycardia if it occurs. **Labetalol** in 2.5-mg increments can be used if the patient is hypertensive and tachycardiac. All the above should be administered intravenously.

G. Verapamil may not be a good choice for the treatment of supraventricular tachycardia if the patient is hypovolemic because of the potential of vasodilatation, which may cause hypotension.

H. If the patient becomes tachycardiac, one's differential diagnosis should include the following:

   1. A hyperthyroid state

   2. Hypovolemia

   3. Fever

   4. Sepsis

   5. Hypoxia

   6. Hypercarbia

   7. Malignant hyperthermia

I. **Nitroprusside** is advantageous as an antihypertensive because it does not significantly dilate the uterine vasculature (1 to 10 μg/kg/minute).

J. **Oxytoxin** should not be infused too rapidly in a hypotensive patient as it may cause further hypotension.

K. One should rule out a trophoblastic embolus if the following symptoms occur: cyanosis, hypotension, tachycardia, decreased pulmonary compliance, or decrease in end-tidal CO_2. One should appropriately support the pulmonary and cardiovascular parameters. A dopamine infusion may be necessary to maintain adequate cardiac output.

L. A baseline blood gas should be obtained before the administration of an anesthetic. If it is abnormal, insert an arterial line for several blood gas determinations.

M. A central line should be placed as well as two large bore intravenous catheters.

N. If the patient shows signs of hypoxia, a pulmonary artery catheter should be placed to determine the hemodynamic profile of the patient so that one may administer the proper anesthetic agent to this patient and to enable one to rationally treat any complications.

SUGGESTED READING

Ackerman WE: Anesthesia considerations for complicated hydatidiform molar pregnancies. *Anesth Rev.* 1984; 7:20.

Twiggs LB. Nonneoplastic complications of molar pregnancy. *Clin Obstet Gynecol.* 1984; 7:665.

37

Anesthetic Considerations for the Patient with Failed Intubation

I. **Incidence.** The incidence of difficult airway and difficult intubation is 1/250 to 1/300 in pregnant patients.

II. **General Considerations.** Failed intubation during induction of cesarean section accounts for 28% of anesthesia deaths and aspiration accounts for 40% of deaths.

III. **Clinical Findings**

  A. Predictive signs of a potentially difficult intubation have been reported by Mallampati and modified by Samsoon and Young.

  B. Four classes of patients are given based on the ease of visualization of intrapharyngeal structures:

MALLAM-PATI	SAMSOON & YOUNG MODIFI-CATION	STRUC-TURES VISIBLE	LARYNGO-SCOPY FINDINGS
Class I	Class I	Soft palate, fauces, uvula	Glottis pillars
Class II	Class II	Soft palate,	Posterior

(continued)

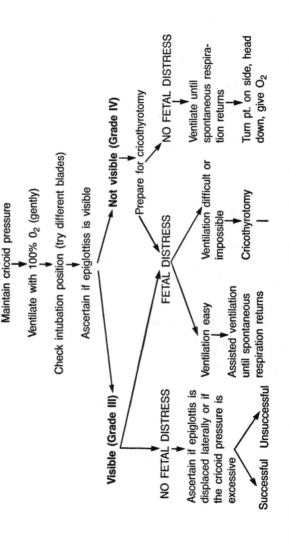

Call for help

Maintain cricoid pressure

Ventilate with 100% O_2 (gently)

Check intubation position (try different blades)

Ascertain if epiglottiss is visible

Visible (Grade III) → NO FETAL DISTRESS → Ascertain if epiglottis is displaced laterally or if the cricoid pressure is excessive → Successful / Unsuccessful

Not visible (Grade IV) → Prepare for cricothyrotomy

FETAL DISTRESS → Ventilation easy → Assisted ventilation until spontaneous respiration returns

FETAL DISTRESS → Ventilation difficult or impossible → Cricothyrotomy

NO FETAL DISTRESS → Ventilate until spontaneous respiration returns → Turn pt. on side, head down, give O_2

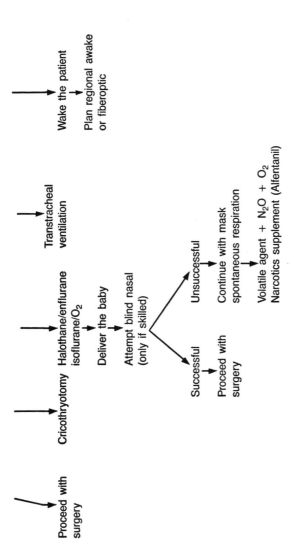

Proceed with surgery

Cricothyrotomy

Transtracheal ventilation

Halothane/enflurane isoflurane/O_2

Deliver the baby

Attempt blind nasal (only if skilled)

Successful → Proceed with surgery

Unsuccessful → Continue with mask spontaneous respiration → Volatile agent + N_2O + O_2 Narcotics supplement (Alfentanil)

Wake the patient

Plan regional awake or fiberoptic

Figure 37–1. Failure to intubate guidelines.

229

MALLAM-PATI	SAMSOON & YOUNG MODIFI-CATION	STRUC-TURES VISIBLE	LARYNGO-SCOPY FINDINGS
		fauces, uvula	commissure
	Class III	Soft palate, base of uvula	Epiglottital tip
Class III	Class IV	Soft palate not visible	No glottal structures visible

IV. Obstetric Management. Skin incision should be delayed until endotracheal intubation has been confirmed or, in the case of life-threatening hemorrhage, when general anesthesia can be accomplished by mask with maintenance of cricoid pressure.

V. Anesthetic Considerations

   A. A failed intubation drill has been described by Tunstall and an algorithm has been described by Shnider and Levinson. A failed intubation protocol should be an essential part of an obstetric anesthesia practice. If one cannot intubate the patient, one must immediately ask for help and use the failed intubation drill as outlined below. The grades are those which were described by Samsoon and Young.

   B. Points to remember

   1. Besides listening for bilateral breath sound, ALWAYS LISTEN TO STOMACH AND TRACHEA for air entry.

   2. Use capnometry and pulse oximetry during the induction of anesthesia.

   3. "When in doubt, take it out."

   4. "Persistence is not a key to success but is a disaster."

> **5.** Attempt to minimize anxiety in the operating room.
>
> **C.** Failure to intubate guidelines (Fig. 37—1)

SUGGESTED READING

Mallampati SR. Clinical sign to predict difficult tracheal intubation. *Can J Anaesth*. 1985; 32:429.

Samsoon GLT, Young JRB. Difficult tracheal intubation. A retrospective study. *Anaesthesia*. 1987; 42:487.

Shnider SM, Levinson G. Anesthesia for Obstetrics. Baltimore: Williams & Wilkins; 1987.

Tunstall ME. Anesthesia for obstetric operations. *Clin Obstet Gynecol*. 1980; 7:665.

38

Anesthetic Considerations for the Patient with Postpartum Tubal Ligation, D&C, and Cerclage

I. Anesthetic Considerations for Bilateral Tubal Ligation

  A. The **advantages** to doing bilateral tubal ligation in the postpartum period are as follows:

    1. An enlarged uterus makes the fallopian tubes easily accessible to the surgeon.

    2. It can be performed with the epidural anesthetic that was used for delivery.

    3. It is a safe and effective means of sterilization, which does not require expensive or complicated equipment.

    4. It can be easily performed immediately postpartum, which reduces the cost of rehospitalization.

  B. Consent forms

    1. A signed sterilization form at the appropriate time during pregnancy needs to be obtained by patient/spouse as required according to hospital/state/federal regulations.

    2. Operative consent form needs to be signed immediately before tubal ligation.

    3. If there is any doubt in the patient's mind concerning the tubal ligation, the procedure should be postponed.

C. Studies regarding postpartum tubal ligations

    1. Blouw et al studied 21 patients, 9 to 42 hours postpartum compared to 11 elective surgical nonpregnant patients and found that 8-hour interval from delivery to anesthetic did not increase risk of aspiration but 33 to 64% of patients in both groups had more than 25 mL of fluid and pH less than 2.5. These patients had general anesthesia.

    2. Uram et al observed that delaying general anesthesia for bilateral tubal ligation more than 2 hours did not improve the patient's safety.

    3. James et al studied three time intervals (1 to 8 hours, 9 to 23 hours, 24 to 45 hours) and found that none of the groups differed from control groups significantly and aspiration risk was high in all groups.

    4. Conclusions of the studies:

        a. The postpartum patient is at a higher risk than the general population.

        b. No safe delivery to surgery interval has been determined.

        c. Preventive measures for aspiration need to be taken.

D. Timing of surgery

    1. It is controversial as to when a postpartum tubal ligation should be performed, either immediately postpartum if the epidural catheter is in place, 6 to 8 hours postdelivery, or within 24 hours.

2. Tubal ligations are elective procedures and since all pregnant patients are considered "full stomachs," general anesthesia is not preferred.

3. If a patient has delivered with a functional epidural, then it seems reasonable to perform a bilateral tubal ligation with that epidural.

4. All patients should receive prophylactic antacids before surgery.

5. A T6 level or higher must be obtained before the incision is made.

6. The epidural catheter may be left in place if surgery cannot be done immediately postpartum. If one anticipates leaving the epdural catheter in place, however, then it must have a sterile dressing applied.

7. If the epidural was not completely functional (ie, partial blockade), then the bilateral tubal ligation should be deferred for 8 hours or until the next day and the patient should be kept NPO during this interval.

E. Anesthetic considerations

1. An increased risk of aspiration is present in the pregnant patient due to mechanical and physiological changes previously discussed but it is not known when gastric emptying returns to normal.

2. Sterilization procedures should not be

performed if there are questions regarding the health of the mother or the neonate (ie, infection, anemia, electrolyte imbalance, and poorly controlled systemic disease).

3. A preoperative anesthetic assessment needs to be obtained to determine that no new medical problems exist.

4. **Laboratory tests:** Postpartum hemoglobin/hematocrit must be done to insure that blood loss during delivery has not been excessive.

5. Premedication is helpful. The dose and type are determined by the anesthetist.

6. One should consider medications that encourage gastric emptying, increase lower esophageal sphincter tone, and neutralize acids (ie, metaclopramide and sodium citrate).

7. Intraoperative monitoring with an ECG, precordial stethoscope, an automated blood pressure cuff, temperature strip, and pulse oximeter must be done.

8. **General anesthesia**
   a. One should do a rapid sequence induction using cricoid pressure and endotracheal intubation.
   b. Choice of agent
      (1) The choice of agent is the preference of the anesthetist.
      (2) The minimum alveolar concentration is decreased with pregnancy.
      (3) One must avoid high inspired concentrations of halogenated agents,

which can decrease uterine contractility.

9. Narcotics: Alfentanyl may be suitable due to the short duration of the procedure and the short duration of action of alfentanyl.

10. Muscle relaxants

    a. Succinylcholine has a short duration of action and is highly ionized. Consequently, minimal quantities reach the breast milk.

    b. Atracurium has a short duration and is easily reversed. Its effect on breast milk is not known, however.

11. Laparoscopic sterilization

    a. Hemodynamic changes associated with peritoneal CO_2 insufflation:

        (1) $PaCO_2$ is increased.

            (a) Carbon dioxide is absorbed through the peritoneal cavity.

            (b) Impairment of ventilation: The Trendelenberg position and increased intra-abdominal distention may make ventilation difficult.

        (2) Insufflation to 20 mm Hg produces stimulation of the cardiovascular (CV) system and the following hemodynamic changes may be seen:

            (a) Increased mean arterial pressure (MAP)

            (b) Increased central venous pressure (CVP)

            (c) Tachycardia

(d) Hypercarbia

(e) Decreased pH

(3) Insufflation to 30 mm Hg produces depression of CV system due to decreased venous return to the heart and the following may be seen:

(a) Decreased CVP

(b) Decreased systolic BP

(c) Decreased pulse pressure

(d) Decreased CO

(4) Cardiac arrhythmias

(a) These patients are more prone to arrhythmias with halothane anesthesia or with the patient breathing spontaneously.

(b) Methods to decrease hemodynamic changes associated with CO_2 insufflation are as follows:

(1) One must not allow intra-abdominal pressure to increase above 20 mm Hg.

(2) One must use atropine or glycopyrrolate to decrease incidence of arrhythmias associated with vasovagal reflexes.

(3) One must use controlled ventilation.

(4) One should avoid the use of halothane due to a lower arrhythmia threshold.

II. Anesthetic Considerations for Dilation and Curettage (D&C)

Abortions are classified clinically as complete, incomplete, or missed. In **complete abortions,** all of the conceptus is expelled. With an **incomplete abortion,** not all of the conceptus is expelled. These patients may have significant bleeding. **Missed abortions** may have decreased fibrogen levels and can bleed. If the patient is hypovolemic, general anesthesia should be considered using ketamine for induction. If the patient's plasma volume is normal, a regional block may be used.

III. Anesthetic Considerations for Cerclage
   A. Etiology. A cerclage is done for cervical incompetence. Cervical incompetence is suggested by a history of repeated second trimester abortions.
   B. The **objective of a cerclage** is as follows:
      1. To prevent effacement and dilatation of cervix.
      2. To prevent fetal loss.
      3. It should be done between the 14th and 18th weeks.
      4. It should be done before cervix is dilated 4 cm.
   C. Contraindications for cerclage are as follows:
      1. Rupture of fetal membranes
      2. Bleeding
      3. Preterm labor
      4. Chorioamnionitis
   D. Type of procedures
      1. Shirodkar procedure:
         a. An incision of vaginal mucosa is made with burying of the suture at the internal os.
         b. If the suture is not removed, a cesarean section may be necessary.

2. McDonald procedure:
   a. This procedure is easier to perform.
   b. The suture is placed superiorly in the body of the cervix near the level of the internal os, followed by continuous placement in the body of the cervix to encircle the os.

E. Anesthetic considerations for cerclage:
   1. The procedure is usually performed at 12 to 14 weeks.
   2. One must consider the possible terato-genetic effects and fetal drug depression related to the anesthetic agents.
   3. One should use local or regional anesthesia if possible. A subarachnoid block exposes the fetus to less local anesthetic mass.
   4. A T10 level is required if a subarachnoid block or epidural is used.
   5. The dose of local anesthetics required during the first and second trimester is not known; an epidural catheter will allow additional dose if required. They should be closely watched in the recovery room after the cerclage has been done.
   6. Patients may require prophylactic tocolytic therapy after the procedure.
   7. If general anesthesia is administered, rapid sequence intubation should be used at 28 weeks' gestation.

SUGGESTED READING

Blouw R, Scatliff J, Palahniuk RJ, et al Gastric volume and pH in postpartum patients. *Anesthesiology*. 1976; 45:456.

Brodsky JB, Cohen EN, Brown BW Jr. et al. Surgery during pregnancy and fetal outcome. *Am J Obstet Gynecol*. 1980; 138:1165.

James CF, Gibbs CP, Banner TE. Postpartum perioperative risk of pulmonary aspiration pneumonia. *Anesthesiology*. 1984; 61:756.

Sidhu MS, Cullen BF. Low dose enflurance does not increase blood loss during therapeutic abortion. *Anesthesiology*. 1982; 57:127.

Uram M, Abouleish E, McKenzie R, et al. The risk of aspiration pneumonitis with postpartum tubal ligation. In: Abstracts of scientific papers. Annual Meeting, Society of Obstetric Anesthesia and Perinatology. Jackson Hole, Wy. 1982.

39

Anesthetic Considerations for Non-Obstetric Surgery During Pregnancy

I. Incidence. The incidence of surgery during pregnancy is 0.3 to 1.6% of all pregnancies.

II. General Considerations

A. Elective major surgery should be avoided during pregnancy.

B. The second trimester is usually the optimal time for operative procedures if they must be done.

C. During the first trimester, hypoxia can cause congenital anomalies in the developing fetus.

D. Abortion following surgery is not common unless uterine manipulation was done intraoperatively or if the patient had peritoneal sepsis.

E. It is estimated that 50,000 pregnant women may receive an anesthetic each year.

F. Surgery during pregnancy is not related to a greater frequency of maternal death than obstetric patients in general.

G. The perinatal mortality is increased.

H. For the safety of the developing fetus, one must avoid any non-emergency surgery if possible.

I. The **most common surgical conditions** are appendicitis and torsion rupture or hemorrhage of ovarian cysts.

    1. The incidence of an ovarian cyst requiring surgery (first and second trimester) is 1:2500.

    2. The incidence of acute appendicitis is 0.07% (most common emergency).

J. **Cholecystectomies** may also be done as gallstones can form because of retardation in the filling and emptying of the gallbladder during pregnancy and because of the increased cholesterol content of the blood, which favors formation of gallstones during pregnancy.

K. The **repair of an incompetent cervix** (Shirodkar and McDonald procedures) may be done in the first and second trimesters (usually after 20 weeks).

L. Other reports of critical conditions with survival during pregnancy include:

    1. Intracranial tumors and aneurysm

    2. Cardiac disease with resulting cardiac surgery

    3. Pheochromocytoma

    4. Hyperthyroidism

M. Trauma may necessitate surgery and general anesthesia during pregnancy.

III. Clinical Findings. Symptoms seen with pregnancy, nausea, vomiting, and abdominal pain may also be caused by a non-obstetric illness.

IV. Obstetric Management. Intraoperatively during abdominal surgery, manipulation of the uterus must be minimal to decrease the risk of premature labor.

V. Anesthetic Considerations

A. Concerns for the anesthetist include:

1. The maternal physiological changes that have been presented in a previous chapter.

2. The adverse effects of drugs on the fetus. The anesthesiologist should try to avoid teratogenic drugs and avoid intrauterine asphyxia. Hypotension must be avoided. One must also be concerned about premature labor. Therefore, the patient should be carefully monitored in the recovery room for uterine contractions.

3. If anesthesia is inadequate during surgery, catecholamine production caused by a painful surgical stimulus could cause vasoconstriction, including uterine artery vasoconstriction, which could decrease uterine perfusion.

B. Maternal physiological changes occur that can influence one's anesthetic management.

1. The pregnant patient is different physiologically as was mentioned previously.

2. The physiological changes that occur are due to hormonal secretions of the corpus luteum and placenta and to mechanical factors of the growing uterus, especially in the second and third trimesters.

3. These hormonal changes alter the patient's physiological response to anesthetic techniques and drugs.

C. Effects of anesthesia on the embryo or fetus, or both:

1. Teratogenicity refers to environmental or genetic effects for producing adverse mor-

phological, biochemical, or behavioral fetal effects.

2. Teratogen will result in a defect if appropriate doses are given or if it is given in the developmental stage or if a specific drug is given to a susceptible species.

3. The greatest periods of sensitivity for the developing organs are as follows:

    a. Heart: 18 to 40 days.

    b. Limbs: 24 to 34 days.

    c. The human brain is vulnerable from the seventh month to the first few months after birth.

4. If fetal damage is generalized, it results in a miscarriage.

5. If fetal damage is localized, it results in congenital anomalies (ie, over 75% of thalidomide patients delivered normal infants).

6. A definite correlation between anesthetic drugs and fetal anomalies has not been established due to the many factors responsible for anomaly production.

    a. Drug exposure is only one factor to take into consideration.

    b. Maternal hypoxemia, hypercarbia, infection, stress, radiation, and malnutrition are other factors that must be taken into consideration.

D. Animal studies

    1. Animal studies are sometimes difficult to interpret because the concentration and duration of anesthetic given is usually far in excess of normal clinical dosages.

    2. Small study populations and lack of controls noted make results of animal studies difficult to interpret.

3. It is difficult to determine which anesthetic is preferable for the first trimester of pregnancy. Those substances, which readily cross placenta, are those with high lipid solubilities and molecular weights lower than 600.

4. One must assume that any anesthetic agent that penetrates the embryo has the potential for producing anomalies until proven otherwse.

5. The applicability of animal studies has not been determined to date.

E. Systemic medications have been studied.

   1. Studies have suggested that an association exists between **minor tranquilizers** during pregnancy and an increased risk of congenital anomalies.

   2. In a study of prenatal records, 19,000 births were reviewed whose mothers had taken **meprobamate** or **chlordiazepoxide,** which showed an increased incidence of anomalies when these medications were prescribed in the first 6 weeks of gestation.

   3. The **Finnish Register of Congenital Malformations** (1967 to 1971) reported an association of cleft palate with the ingestion of diazepam and meprobamate, salicylates, and opiates.

   4. Mothers with infants with cleft lips, with or without cleft palates, reported the use of diazepam four times more frequently

than mothers of infants with other defects. Phenytoin may also cause anomalies.

5. A study of more than 50,000 human pregnancies with 1300 mothers with various doses of phenothiozine during the first 4 months of pregnancy showed no adverse effects on perinatal mortality, birth weight, congenital abnormalities, or IQ scores at 4 years of age.

6. The FDA reported in September, 1985, "While these data do not provide conclusive evidence that minor tranquilizers cause fetal abnormalities, they do suggest an association. Since the use of these drugs during the first trimester of pregnancy is rarely a matter of urgency, benefit/risk considerations are such that their use during this period should almost always be avoided."

7. With reference to narcotics, hypoxia and hypercarbia induced by narcotics are responsible for teratogenic effect rather than the narcotics themselves.

F. Anesthetics:

1. **N_2O** is the most extensively studied.
   a. In rats, 50% N_2O resulted in a high incidence of intrauterine death and increased skeletal malformations.
   b. In chicken eggs exposed to 80% N_2O, those that hatched had a high degree of neurological defects.

2. **Halothane** can cause anomalies in the rat fetus. Cleft palates and paw defects were reported in mice. Increased abortions

midgestation were reported in hamsters.

3. Muscle relaxants cross the placenta to some extent. It used to be felt that they did not cross the placenta due to increased ionization and low lipid solubility. There is no evidence that normal clinical doses have any adverse effects on human fetal development.

4. With reference to local anesthetics:
   a. Blood levels reach the fetus in low levels following subarachnoid block.
   b. Blood levels following epidural administration or inadvertent intravascular injection may be very high.
   c. Bupivacaine and etidocaine injected into rabbits and rats did not demonstrate teratogenecity.

5. Human studies
   a. Very few studies were done for obvious ethical reasons. It is difficult to say that anesthesia does not cause teratogenecity. Those studies done to date have not shown an increase in fetal anomalies.
   b. No anesthetic appears itself to be a potent teratogen.
   c. Studies in the United States and Great Britain suggested that female anesthesiologists and wives of male anesthetists may have an increased rate of abortion.
   d. Shnider and Webster reviewed 147 women (47 first trimester, 58 second trimester, and 42 third trimester) who received anesthesia during pregnancy

(Shnider, 1965). They were compared to 8926 who delivered at this time. The incidence of anomalies was not significantly different.

6. Ventilation

a. In experimental animals, hyperoxia, hypoxia, and hypercapnia may be teratogenic.

b. Congenital anomalies have been reported after exposure to hypoxia in rats, rabbits, mice, and chicks.

c. The effects of hyperoxia are debatable.

d. Chronic hypoxemia is not associated with increased incidence of anomalies.

e. Behavioral teratology: Currently there is no evidence that has established that anesthesia adversely affects the mental and neurological development in infants.

f. One must avoid **intrauterine fetal asphyxia.**

  (1) The uteroplacental circulation is indirectly and easily affected by drugs and anesthesia procedures.

  (2) **Fetal oxygenation** depends on the following:

   (a) Maternal oxygenation; therefore, one must avoid hypoxic situations (ie, laryngospasm, airway obstruction, low inspired oxygen).

   (b) One must be concerned about oxygen delivery and therefore the hemoglobin.

  (3) Uteroplacental perfusion is de-

creased by maternal hypotension, hypertension, hemorrhage, regional anesthesia, and aortocaval compression. Regional anesthesia, however, can correct decreases in uteroplacental perfusion caused by pregnancy-induced hypertension.

(4) Increased uterine activity may also result in uteroplacental perfusion. One must avoid the use of alpha-adrenergic drugs. Ketamine, greater than 1 mg/kg, also increases uterine tone.

(5) Administration of epinephrine and norepinephrine can also decrease uteroplacental perfusion. Ephedrine is the drug of choice for hypotension.

7. Premature labor
   a. Premature labor should be avoided.
   b. No study has shown that any one agent or technique has been found to be associated with a higher or lower incidence of premature labor.
   c. It seems to be related to surgical pathology and manipulation, especially in pelvic organs.

G. In summary, during pregnancy, only emergency surgery should be performed. Elective procedures should be delayed until physiological changes have returned to normal. When doing a preoperative assessment for all childbearing women, one must always check for possible pregnancy.

H. Emergency surgery
  1. One must preoxygenate and do a rapid sequence intubation if a general anesthetic must be done. A non-particulate antacid (15 to 30 ML sodium citrate) should be given before the induction of anesthesia.
  2. At the beginning of the second trimester, avoid the supine position. One must use the lateral position or left uterine displacement to decrease the risk of aortocaval compression.
  3. One should monitor the fetal heart rate after the 16th week as well as monitoring the fetus postoperatively.

 I. When doing regional anesthesia, one must avoid hypotension, preload each patient with lactated Ringer's (20 mL/kg), decrease the dose of local anesthetics by one third, use left uterine displacement, avoid maternal blood pressure, and, if a vasopressor is required, one must use ephedrine (10 to 25 mg IV) in 5-mg increments.

J. If general anesthesia must be administered:
  1. A preoperative evaluation must be done.
  2. Preoxygenation should be done on every patient.
  3. Rapid controlled induction with cricoid pressure must be maintained until the endotracheal cuff is inflated.
  4. Hypoxemic episodes must be avoided.
  5. During the first trimester, one must use drugs that have had a safe history. The following drugs may be used:
     a. Thiopental, up to 4 mg/kg.
     b. Fentanyl.

    c. Succinylcholine, d-tubocurare, and Pavulon.

    d. Low concentration of N_2O.

    e. Halothane, enflurane, or isoflurane offers the advantage of decreased uterine tone and may be helpful.

  6. Maternal hyperventilation must be avoided. A capnometer should be used.

  7. Blood gases must be monitored routinely on long cases. The maternal PaO_2 must be maintained between 100 and 200 torr, while the Pco_2 should be kept at 30 torr.

K. In the recovery room, one should do the following:

  1. A pulse oximeter should be used to assess oxygenation.

  2. Vital signs must be maintained. Hypotension should be vigorously treated.

  3. Fetal and uterine monitoring should be done on all patients postoperatively.

  4. The patient must be extubated awake.

  5. In the recovery room, if analgesics must be given, the minimal effective doses of narcotics should be administered. Epidural analgesia may be of benefit in the postoperative period.

SUGGESTED READING

Brodsky JB, Cohen EN, Brown BW, Jr., et al. Surgery during pregnancy and fetal outcome. *Am J Obstet Gynecol*. 1980; 138:1165.

Duncan PG, Pope WDB, Cohen MM, et al. Fetal risk of anesthesia and surgery during pregnancy. *Anesthesiology*. 1986; 64:790.

Levinson G, Shnider SM, de LoRimier AA, et al. Effects of maternal hyperventilation on uterine blood flow and fetal oxygenation and acid base status. *Anesthesiology*. 1974; 40:340.

Shnider SM, Webster GM. Maternal and fetal hazards of surgery during pregnancy. *Am J Obstet Gynecol*. 1965; 92:891.

40

Anesthetic Considerations for the Patient Undergoing In Vitro Fertilization

I. In vitro fertilization consists of the harvesting of a mature oocyte by laparoscopy. Once the oocyte is harvested, it is transferred to an external medium and exposed to a sperm where fertilization occurs. Following fertilization, the fertilized egg is returned to the uterine cavity for maturation. Local, regional, and general anesthesia have all been used for laparoscopy for in vitro fertilization.

A. Anesthetic considerations. Stress or uterine contractions may each have a physiological effect on the successful placement of a human conceptus. Uterine contractions can cause expulsion of the human conceptus. It has been suggested that halothane may interfere with the oocyte membrane and with polyspermy. Data by Nuccitelli et al have shown that halothane inhibits sperm motility, and it has therefore been reported that halothane should be avoided as an anesthetic agent during gamete intrafallopian transfer (GIFT). Consequently, one may want to consider the use of either enflurane or isoflurane during laparoscopy with a muscle relaxant to prevent a patient from moving.

B. Epidural analgesia. Epidural anesthesia has been used for gynecologic laparoscopy. The duration of laparoscopy for oocyte retrieval is relatively long, however, and, in a published report by Lehtinen et al, only 3 of 11 patients were completely without pain during the procedure. The problems associated with epidural anesthesia are pain during surgical manipulation, the steep Trendelenburg position, and the insufflation of the peritoneum with carbon dioxide, which can make spontaneous ventilation for patients very difficult.

C. Subarachnoid anesthesia. If general anesthesia cannot be used, a suitable alternative method is subarachnoid anesthesia. It has been shown by Endler to be a safe and efficacious alternative to general anesthesia in instances where general anesthesia was not indicated.

II. Complications

A. Cardiac complications. During laparoscopy, hypotension and decreases in cardiac output can occur secondary to the pneumoperitoneum and the resulting increased intrabdominal pressure following insufflation, which can reduce venous return. At the conclusion of the procedure, the patient should be returned slowly to the horizontal position from the Trendelenburg position to decrease the incidence of hypotension.

B. Pulmonary complications. The steep Trendelenburg position and the pneumoperitoneum can reduce a patient's vital capacity. One must, therefore, observe the patients for the incidence of postoperative respiratory complications, including pneumomediastinum. A gas embolus or a pneumothorax related to the retroperitoneal dissection of carbon dioxide during insufflation may be observed on occasion. One might suspect either of these complications if cyanosis and hypotension suddenly occur.

C. Hemorrhage. Trauma to blood vessels can occur during the laparoscopy procedure. Bleeding can range from minor bleeding from trauma to superficial vessels, or may be manifest as massive hemorrhage caused by laceration of major retroperitoneal blood vessels. If sudden hypotension occurs intraoperatively, one must ask the obstetrician if bleeding is observed through the laparoscope.

SUGGESTED READING

Endler GC. Use of spinal anesthesia in laparoscopy for in vitro fertilization. *Fertil Steril.* 1985; 43:809.

Fishel S. General anesthesia for intrauterine placement of human conceptuses after in vitro fertilization. *J In Vitro Fertil Embryo Transfer.* 1987; 4:260.

Hayes NF. Effect of general anesthesia on fertilization and cleavage of human oocytes in vitro. *Fertil Steril.* 1987; 48:975.

Lehtinen A. Modifying effects of epidural analgesia or general anesthesia on the stress hormone response to laparoscopy for in vitro fertilization. *J In Vitro Fertil Embryo Transfer.* 1987; 4:23.

Nuccitelli R. Controversy over the fast partial temporary blocked polyspermi in sea urchins: A reevaluation. *Dev Biol.* 1984; 1:103.

SECTION IX

Appendices

Appendix A

Laboratory Values of Concern in Pregnancy

	Nonpregnant Female	Pregnant Female
White blood cells	4500–11,000/μL	15,000/μL; in labor, up to 25,000/μL
Platelets	200,000–400,000 μL	200,000–400,000 μL
Hemoglobin	12–16 g/dL	>10 g/dL[a]
Hematocrit	37–47%	>30%[a]
Fibrinogen level	150–300 mg/dL	250–600 mg/dL (in second and third trimesters)
Bleeding time (Ivy)	No difference (1–7 min)	
Erythrocyte sedimentation rate (Wintrobe scale)	0–20 mm/h	Increases 2–6 times the nonpregnant values
Fasting glucose	65–96 mg/dL	65–110 mg/dL
Serum albumin	3.5–5.0 g/dL	3.5–6.0 g/dL at term
Transaminases		
SGOT	8–20 mU/mL	8–20 mU/mL
SGPT	8–20 U/L	8–20 U/L
LDH	45–100 U/L	May be increased
Bilirubin		
Total	<0.2–1.0 mg/dL	<0.2–1.0 mg/dL
Direct	<0.2 mg/dL	<0.2 mg/dL
Indirect	<0.8 mg/dL	<0.8 mg/dL
Blood urea nitrogen	7–18 mg/dL	7–9 mg/dL

(continued)

	Nonpregnant Female	Pregnant Female
Creatinine	0.6–1.1 mg/dL	0.4–0.58 mg/dL
Urine		
pH	4.6–8.0	Acid
Glucose	Negative	Glucosuria can be normal
Protein	Negative	Proteinuria can be common

[a]Dilutional anemia of pregnancy.

Appendix B

Common Obstetric Terms and Abbreviations

Terms Commonly Used in Obstetrics

1. Contractions of true labor
   a. Regular intervals are present.
   b. The intervals gradually shorten.
   c. The intensity gradually increases.
   d. Cervix dilates.
2. Cervical effacement
   a. Expressed in terms of the length of the cervical canal.
   b. When the length is reduced by one half, it is 50% effaced.
   c. When it becomes as thin as the lower uterine segment, it is 100% effaced.
3. Station (+3 cm to −3 cm)
   a. When the lowermost portion of the presenting part of the fetal head is at the level of the ischial spine, it is at zero station.
   b. When the head is above the level of the ischial spine, it is said to be at minus station.
4. Lie: Lie is the relationship of the long axis of the fetus in relation to the long axis of the mother. Normally, the lie of the fetus is longitudinal.

5. Dilatation (0—10 cm): Describes the magnitude of the opening of the cervical os.
6. Presentation
   a. Defines the part of the fetus that is lowermost in the pelvis.
   b. Normal presentation is vertex.

Abbreviations Commonly Used in Obstetrics

AROM	Artificial rupture of membranes—amniotomy
BAL	Ballottable—head is engaged
BR	Breech
BTL	Bilateral tubal ligation
C/S	Cesarean section
CST	Contraction stress test
DM	Diabetes mellitus
EDC	Expected date of confinement (due date)
FHR/FHT	Fetal heart rate or tones
Gest DM	Gestational diabetes mellitus
ID	Induction-delivery time (time pentothal is administered until cord is clamped)
INC AB	Incomplete abortion
Irreg	Irregular uterine contraction pattern
IUFD	Intrauterine fetal death
IUP	Intrauterine pregnancy
LNMP	Last normal menstrual period
L/S ratio	Lechithin sphingomyelin ratio (used to determine fetal lung maturity)
Mec	Meconium
$MgSO_4$	Magnesium sulfate
NCB	Natural childbirth

NIL	Not in labor
NST	Non-stress test
OCT	Oxytocin challenge test
PIH	Pregnancy-induced hypertension
PIT	Pitocin
PROM	Premature rupture of membranes
SROM	Spontaneous rupture of membranes
TAB	Therapeutic abortion
TOL	Trial of labor in previous cesarean section
UD	Uterine delivery time (time uterus incised until cord is clamped)
VBAC	Vaginal birth after cesarean section

Index